Bowel Cancer
Foundations for Practice

Edited by **Barbara Borwell** MA(ED), RGN, DIP COUNSELLING

Specialist Nurse Consultant/Associate Lecturer, Institute of Health
and Community Studies, Bournemouth University

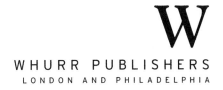

WHURR PUBLISHERS
LONDON AND PHILADELPHIA

© 2005 Whurr Publishers Ltd
First published 2005
by Whurr Publishers Ltd
19b Compton Terrace
London N1 2UN England and
325 Chestnut Street, Philadelphia PA 19106 USA

British Library Cataloguing in Publication Data

A catalogue record for this book
is available from the British Library.

ISBN 1 86156 452 X

Typeset by Adrian McLaughlin, a@microguides.net
Printed and bound in the UK by Athenæum Press Limited, Gateshead, Tyne & Wear

Contents

Foreword

Thirteen years ago, when I was presenter of the BBC's *Watchdog* programme, I was diagnosed with advanced bowel cancer after nearly a year of medical delay. I had never heard of the disease – I had no idea that it was the second biggest cancer killer in the UK and, a decade later, set to become the most common cancer across Europe.

I welcome this book and urge health professionals to read it for the support that it will give you both in understanding this dreadful disease and in your efforts to help us, your patients, at whatever stage of our journey to survive it, live with it, die from it with understanding and dignity.

Lynn Faulds-Wood
September 2004

Preface

Bowel (or colorectal) cancer is a significant health problem of the twenty-first century. On a worldwide scale, it is the fourth most common cancer, associated with substantial morbidity and mortality (Boyle, 1998).

For a health-care system to meet the demands of a patient suffering from bowel cancer, it is vital that a good working relationship is established between those engaged in the different aspects of care.

Development of readers' knowledge and skills in both theory and practice will enable nurses to demonstrate knowledge acquisition and understanding of the challenges posed by cancer in their area of nursing practice. This increased awareness will provide opportunities for nurses to develop strategies that can further enhance the quality and effectiveness of patient care.

Having worked in the field of specialist nursing for over 20 years, with the major component being in the field of cancer care, I have a total commitment to patient-focused care and multidisciplinary team working. My involvement in oncology nurse education reflects these principles and provides opportunities to utilize past experience, and current and political debate for the benefit of nursing practice.

The purpose of this book is to provide a comprehensive introduction to bowel cancer for all health professionals involved in the care of these patients and their families, empowering patients to cope with the challenges newly imposed by a cancer diagnosis, supported by a multiprofessional team with a shared commitment to maximizing the quality of the patient's experience.

This book has been designed and written to assist the reader in embarking on a bowel cancer journey from its evolution and treatment, to patient- and family-centred care including consideration of an individual's social, spiritual and psychological needs, in either the hospital or the community setting.

The contributors to this volume reflect this philosophy, and bring together a wealth of experience and specialist knowledge, thus providing a concise and readable foundation on which to base current health-care practice.

Barbara Borwell

Reference

Boyle P (1998) Some recent developments in the epidemiology of colorectal cancer. In: Bleiberg H, Rougier P, Wilkie HJ (eds), Management of Colorectal Cancer. London: Martin Dunitz.

Acknowledgements

I am indebted to all the contributors. In spite of all their other commitments they have endeavoured to meet the deadlines and share their expertise. Thanks to Lynne Baker, Juliet Borwell, Janet Hick and Gordon Hunt for support and 'technical know-how', and those anonymous reviewers for their encouragement and useful remarks.

Contributors

Rose Amey BSc, DipSW, DipHE, PQSW Accredited Practice Teacher in Social Work, Oncology/Haematology Social Worker, Dorset County Hospital, Dorchester

Tanya Andrewes RGN, BSc(Hons), PGDipEd, Senior Lecturer, Institute of Health and Community Studies, Bournemouth University, Bournemouth

Barbara Borwell MA(Ed), RGN, NDN, BCN, Dip Counselling, Cert Psychosexual Counselling and Therapy, Specialist Nurse Consultant/Associate Lecturer, Institute of Health and Community Studies, Bournemouth University, Bournemouth

Helena Bridgman MSc, RGN, RSCN, Senior Nurse Manager for Specialist Palliative Care, Salisbury; Lead Cancer Nurse for Salisbury Healthcare NHS Trust, Salisbury

Ian Donaldson BEd, MA, DipN, RNT, RN, Senior Lecturer, Bournemouth University, Bournemouth

Wendy Farrell BSc(Hons), RN, Community Cancer Nurse Specialist, Poole Primary Care Trust and Lecturer/Practitioner affiliated to Bournemouth University, Bournemouth

Helen Gandhi RGB, SCM, Dip Counselling, Dip Counselling and Professional Development, Dip Aromatherapy, Dip Reflexology, Psychodynamic Independent Clinical Nurse Specialist, Colorectal and Stoma Care

Catherine Hughes BSc(Hons), RGN, DipN, Community Cancer Nurse Specialist, Poole Primary Care Trust and Lecturer/Practitioner affiliated to Bournemouth University, Bournemouth

Barry Rawlings BSc, MA(Ed), PGCEA, RGN, DipN, Nursing Lecturer, Institute of Health and Community Studies, Bournemouth University, Bournemouth

Barbara Stuchfield RGN, Senior CNS Colorectal/Stoma Care, St Bartholomew's and the London NHS Trust

Emily Walters BSc(Hons), State-Registered Dietitian, Lead Dietitian, Cancer Centre, Southampton University Hospital Trust, Southampton

Introduction

Helena Bridgman

Between 1985 and 1989, a comparison of cancer survival rates across 17 European countries, using data collected from both national and regional registries, was conducted (Eurocare Study: WHO, IARC, EC 1995). This indicated that outcomes of care in the UK were poor despite an advanced health-care economy. A further study comparing outcomes of care specifically for colorectal cancer patients in the western world (Cancer Research Campaign 1999) also demonstrated significant differences in 5-year survival between the whole of Europe (47%) and the UK (40.9%).

It is important to consider methodological differences in data collection when using international comparisons to distinguish between what is reality and what may be artefact (Woodman et al. 2001), but substantial evidence remains that the most recent data for England and Wales demonstrate that over 30 000 individuals are diagnosed with colorectal cancer per annum, many of whom present with advanced disease (Quinn et al. 2001). In addition, about half of these patients will die of their disease whereas survival rates are now between 40.9 and 45% at 5 years after diagnosis (National Cancer Guidance Steering Group or NCGSG 2004). Identified reasons for this have been multiple but have included ignorance of risk factors or fear of their implication, delays in communication between primary and secondary care, timeliness and national parity of investigations and treatment regimens, and equity of access to supportive and palliative care.

The challenge for government health policy and the multidisciplinary teams that directly deliver care in the twenty-first century has been to develop a framework that reduces inequalities in cancer care. This is being achieved by providing service models based on locally identified needs' assessment and evidence-based treatment guidance, and the redesign of existent services to improve cure rates and quality of life for all individuals with a diagnosis of colorectal cancer.

Historical background

The Calman–Hine Report (Expert Advisory Group on Cancer 1995) set the agenda for significant organizational and cultural change, which continues to evolve within the context of The NHS Cancer Plan (Department of Health or DoH 2000b) and improving outcomes guidance (IOG). This, the first of the National Service Frameworks, prioritized continuity and coordination of cancer care through the creation of managed clinical networks charged with providing patient-centred services. For the first time, service commissioners and providers, voluntary organizations and local authorities would work as a team to provide 'seamless' care throughout the patient cancer journey, from diagnosis to cure or into palliative care. They would develop joint service delivery plans which exercised a consensus when identifying and funding common resource needs and creating solutions for filling perceived gaps in service provision.

These teams would be representative of an integrated three-tier structure of care led by primary care and supported by secondary and tertiary care. Primary care would be responsible for the rapid referral of individuals with a suspected cancer and would manage the day-to-day care of patients in their own homes, where most individuals spend most of their time while living with cancer and its effects. The most common cancers, which include colorectal cancer, would be treated in secondary care cancer units, usually district general hospitals, by teams with sufficient expertise and facilities. The final level of care would be provided by tertiary care cancer centres, for both common and less common cancers, which would also provide specialist diagnostic and therapeutic techniques, such as radiotherapy, to support the local clinical teams. Crucially, for outcomes of care to improve, it would be necessary for all teams to receive appropriate and ongoing training in cancer- and site-specific care in order to provide clinically effective care based on the most up-to-date research evidence.

In 1997, the NHS Clinical Outcomes Group (COG) published the clinical outcomes guidance for colorectal cancer. This guidance acknowledged that, although there was a growing body of scientific evidence to generate improvements in colorectal/bowel cancer outcomes, uncertainty remained in many areas of care. These included the effectiveness of population screening and existent follow-up, and whether cancer of the colon and cancer of the rectum required care under different clinical and organizational structures as a result of the complexity and associated morbidity of surgical interventions for the latter. It was also acknowledged that the vagueness of presenting symptoms meant that many colorectal cancer patients either presented as emergencies with associated morbidity or were referred by a variety of routes, which could cause significant delays in treatment. The quality and availability of diagnostic services were known to be variable and existent clinical practice needed review using targeted clinical trials to clarify the most effective future treatment modalities. Crucially, qualitative outcomes relating to the patient's experience of care needed to be identified. The IOG (NHS Clinical Outcomes Group 1997, updated to NICE 2004) demonstrated that much of the original content is valid but there have been a few important areas of new evidence and the 2004 edition now includes the management of anal cancer as a separate entity.

The implications of the IOG for existing teams could not and cannot be overestimated because, despite achievements to date, more remains to be done. Care delivery based on performance targets places all individuals under the spotlight because a core requirement continues to be the need for audit, to establish which teams are achieving the best care outcomes and whether 'fitness to provide services' should be based on recorded outcomes and a stated minimum level of service activity. Accurate retrospective data have been hard to clarify using an information technology (IT) infrastructure which has been the victim of chronic under-investment, so original figures have been at best arbitrary but have still been used in some cases to make significant changes in the way teams work and relate to specialist centres. The interpretation of the IOG has caused controversy within some local teams with its potential to undermine the practice of senior skilled clinicians, however unintentionally. This unfortunate aspect of its impact has threatened the key to successful organizational change, namely collaborative working and partnership between all providers of care.

The appointment of a National Cancer Director in 1999 sent a clear signal that cancer would be a top priority within the government's modernization agenda for the NHS, presented in The NHS Plan (DoH 2000a). This was closely followed in September 2000 by the publication of The NHS Cancer Plan (DoH 2000b) and the appointment of a Cancer Taskforce to oversee its implementation. This 10-year comprehensive strategy, building on the foundations set by The Calman–Hine Report (Expert Advisory Group on Cancer 1995), aimed to improve the survival and quality of life of all cancer patients, with the target of reducing the death rate from cancer in people under 75 years by at least a fifth by 2010, to compare with the best outcomes in Europe. Advances and service improvements were to be made in the patient cancer journey, through prevention, screening, diagnosis, treatment, supportive and palliative care. This would be achieved by tackling health inequalities, providing clinically effective treatments with equal access to them nationwide, and also, uncommonly for a politically driven vehicle, to plan long term by investing in an infrastructure that would sustain a sufficient and knowledgeable workforce, supported by the latest equipment.

Underpinning all this was the priority to be given to the patient experience, which would influence the redesign of services and the creation of new roles. The Cancer Services Collaborative, more recently known as the Cancer Services Collaborative Service Improvement Partnership (CSC 'IP'), was to spearhead this, bringing 'users' of cancer services, represented by patients, carers, managers and health professionals, together in Partnership Groups to examine the systems by which care was currently delivered. The patient cancer journey would be 'mapped' to aid communication and patient satisfaction with services, prioritizing patient preference and informed decision-making; the plan was to change ways of working to prevent duplication of workload that sometimes leads to significant time delays, and to develop new roles to provide dedicated expertise, availability and consistency in care delivery.

There are now 37 clinically managed cancer networks in place. These work alongside the CSC 'IP' and Partnership Groups, with the aim of delivering consistent levels of care across primary, secondary and tertiary settings. There is an inevitability that, in a health service that delivers care free at the point of delivery, the challenge in making the patient choice agenda a reality and understanding what that really means to the individual will continue to grow because pragmatism vies with idealism in a cash-strapped health economy. However, it has been clear that some changes in service delivery have not been costly. The results of the National Cancer Survey (Airey et al. 2002) found that most patients reported very positively on their experience of care, but access to both clear and accurate written and verbal information about their condition, and also a named professional who could promote continuity of care, were identified as immediate priorities. Information pathways, integrated care pathways and the evolving role of nurse-led services are all examples of significant patient-driven developments and the first national Peer Review of Cancer Services in 2001–2 recognized the many improvements that had been made in services for colorectal cancer patients. Work, however, still remains to be done in standardizing and improving the provision of appropriately trained staff and resources across the country, at all stages of the patient pathway.

Opportunities and challenges for the multidisciplinary team

One of the major objectives in compiling Bowel Cancer: Foundations for Practice has been to provide a review of the contribution of the multidisciplinary team (MDT) to patient management and care outcomes and of the developments allied to the implementation of The NHS Cancer Plan, following the patient through defined stages of the cancer journey.

Facilitating changes in health-related behaviours to reduce the risk of developing colorectal cancer are key to improving survival rates and form the basis of the National Service Framework for Cancer. The implementation of primary preventive strategies, such as Bowel Cancer Awareness Month and the UK's leading colorectal cancer charity, Colon Cancer Concern, is a complex process where an individual's freedom to access help has psychological, social and environmental factors. In a health service that has often been accused of being a 'sickness service' driven by the financial demands placed on secondary care, this requires a major shift in culture as well as training and support for health professionals to promote changes in lifestyle and attitudes. The comprehensive guidance on cancer prevention produced by the Health Development Agency (2002) gives direction to primary care trusts and their cancer leads, together with their partners, in the strategic planning and delivery of cancer services, because the guidance can be interpreted in the context of local needs, resources and circumstances. Changes to the GP contract, which include rewards for services tailored to the local community, may also benefit areas of deprivation or where special needs have been identified.

For outcomes to improve, earlier detection of colorectal cancer not only will be dependent on raising public awareness, but will also require targeted secondary prevention for high-risk and at-risk groups. This has significant implications for future workforce planning and training to meet the increased demand for screening techniques. Inconclusive data resulting from the national screening pilots for detecting colorectal cancer have led to a further option appraisal, which has serious implications for already stretched and under-resourced services, but may herald opportunities for new and advanced practice roles (DoH 1999). In October 2003, it was announced that three national and seven regional endoscopy training centres will train nurses, GPs and allied health professionals (AHPs) in endoscopic procedures, as the focus of diagnostic effort moves from barium enemas to endoscopy. This is one example of the potential for innovation in cancer care roles and responsibilities, which continues to evolve.

Rapid and accurate diagnosis and care of cancer patients, with a maximum 2-month wait from urgent referral to commencement of treatment cited for all cancers by 2008, except for sound clinical reasons or through patient choice, will rely on proactive primary and secondary prevention, robust systems for tracking referrals and a workforce to support this. Systems should also be in place for emergency patients (particularly those with intestinal obstruction) to be promptly referred to and managed by colorectal cancer MDTs. Efficacy of care will rely on the streamlining of services led by the MDT, a growing evidence base for effective drugs and technologies that will be available wherever the patient is treated, national datasets that will inform on the process and outcomes of care, and monitoring of progress, based on regular peer review. Controversy and ethical debate now centre on the knock-on effect that these developments may have on patients with illnesses other than cancer, with the potential for delays in timely treatments. There is also the potential for tensions to develop as the different National Service Frameworks compete for limited resources and achievement of performance indicators. Only time and accurate data will clarify the reality of these concerns.

Ironically, the greatest challenge facing the health professional will probably be directly associated with the drive to improve outcomes. The increasing knowledge base and availability of treatments mean that individuals requiring supportive and palliative care are now generally living longer, often with complex problems in the community. The Supportive and Palliative Care Guidance (National Institute for Clinical Excellence or NICE 2004) defines service models in 12 topic areas which will be needed to ensure that patients, their families and their carers live as well as possible with the effects of their illness from pre-diagnosis and treatment, to cure, continuing illness or death and into bereavement. The key message is that delivery of high-quality care is the responsibility of all and promotes the importance of a partnership approach. What this means in reality is a collective responsibility to undertake a baseline assessment of existent services, a gap analysis leading to short-, medium- and long-term actions dependent on local needs and ongoing research and evaluation of the proposed service models. In primary care, the Gold Standards Framework (Thomas 2003), and in secondary care the Integrated Care Pathway for Care of the Dying (Ellershaw and Ward 2003), are two initiatives that are working towards filling gaps in the consistency of multiprofessional care. For the patient with colorectal cancer, reliant on both specialist and generic support services, coordinated care tailored to meet individual needs will contribute to bringing cancer services up to the levels experienced elsewhere in Europe.

Vision for the future

As cancer continues to be the UK's biggest killer, with one in three people diagnosed and one in four people dying from cancer, 60% of patients will continue to be cared for in the community or generic settings in secondary care (Royal College of Nursing or RCN 2003). A major challenge highlighted by the most recent National Cancer Guidance Steering Group

(NCGSG) (NICE 2004) is the timely delivery of an evolving evidence base within a health-care culture marked by rapid changes. Expansion of investigations such as lower gastrointestinal screening and diagnostic services, advanced treatments and qualitative care interventions, which have not only been proven to be the most effective but are affordable, provide a wealth of opportunities for innovations in workforce development.

Provision of cancer training for all health professionals is crucial to support the implementation of The NHS Cancer Plan and the future development of a skilled workforce with identified career pathways and competencies. The composition and function of MDTs need to be reviewed in the light of revised cancer quality measures (Cancer Action Team 2004) which now replace the National Cancer Standards (DoH 2001). These measures highlight the increasing importance of the site-specialist nurse as a key worker and core member of the MDT and the new role development of an MDT coordinator. Both these individuals will have an active role in MDT discussions, reviewing their operational links with specialist centres as reconfiguration of services continues. These developments demonstrate the value of a collective approach that understands and respects roles, allowing the constructive challenge of care decisions and ethical debate with a patient focus. Targeted training in modern techniques, such as the National MDT – Total Mesorectal Excision (MDT – TME) courses will inevitably increase alongside a developing evidence base, demonstrated by the recognition of TME as essential to all aspects of management of the rectal cancer patient (DoH 2004).

Most GPs will see only an average of eight or nine new cancer patients each year. Action continues to be needed to improve recognition of potential colorectal cancer symptoms for rapid endoscopy referral, so training requirements to match the rapid referral criteria specific to each cancer site should be identified and delivered with regular updates and feedback. The Royal College of Nursing has also called for cancer training to extend to all pre-registration nurse education programmes supported by guidelines and frameworks for competencies that link to an identified career pathway (RCN 2003). This follows on from the Nursing Contribution to Cancer Care (DoH 2000c), which focuses on quality issues needed to develop and maintain a skilled nursing and AHP workforce, including education and continuing professional development, recruitment and retention, leadership and management of cancer care.

The National Cancer Research Institute (NCRI), a virtual body representative of leading cancer institutions and charities, now coordinates research initiatives, working with the Cancer Research Networks to use clinical trials data to inform future research directions. This body will have a major role in leading research into cancer genetics. The possibility of cancer prevention and oral cancer treatments should not be underestimated and it is likely that primary care will take a lead in this developing field, reflecting the original focus for care in The Calman–Hine Report. The role of the clinical nurse specialist in this area is already proving to be effective in providing cancer counselling skills, which allow individuals to make informed decisions about their future health care. It also promises considerable potential for development of new roles working with families with susceptibility to inherited cancers (CNO Bulletin 2003).

Over the next couple of years, the National Audit Office will be evaluating the progress of The NHS Cancer Plan against the seven 'Ps'. It will be assessing the success of partnership working, the development of new professional roles and strategies for illness prevention, patient access to care and the degree of patient choice through performance targets and peer review. The chapters in this book demonstrate how MDTs are rising to these challenges.

References

Airey C, Becher H, Erens R et al. (2002) The National Survey of NHS Patients – Cancer: National Overview 1999-2000. London: Department of Health.

Cancer Action Team (2004) The Manual for Cancer Services. London: Department of Health.

Cancer Research Campaign (CRC) (1999) CRC Stats: Large bowel. London: CRC.

CNO Bulletin (2003) Role of Nurses in Genetics Strategy. London: Department of Health.

Department of Health (1999) Making a Difference: Ten key roles for nurses. London: HMSO.

Department of Health (2000a) The NHS Plan. London: HMSO.

Department of Health (2000b) The NHS Cancer Plan: A plan for investment, a plan for reform. London: HMSO.

Department of Health (2000c) The Nursing Contribution to Cancer Care: A strategic programme of action in support of the national cancer programme. London: HMSO.

Department of Health (2001) Manual of Cancer Services Assessment Standards. London: HMSO.

Department of Health (2004) Cancer Quality Measures. London: HMSO.

Ellershaw J, Ward C (2003) Clinical Review: Care of the dying patient: the last hours or days of life. British Medical Journal 326: 30-4.

Expert Advisory Group on Cancer (1995) The Calman-Hine Report: A policy framework for commissioning cancer services. London: Department of Health.

Health Development Agency (2002) Cancer Prevention: A resource to support local action in delivering the NHS Cancer Plan. London: HDA.

National Cancer Guidance Steering Group (2004) Improving Outcomes in Colorectal Cancer. Manual update. London: NICE.

NHS Clinical Outcomes Group (1997) Guidance on Commissioning Cancer Services: Improving outcomes in colorectal cancer. London: Department of Health.

NICE (2004) Supportive and Palliative Care Guidance. London: Department of Health.

Quinn M, Babb P, Brock A et al. (2001) Cancer Trends in England and Wales 1950-1999. London: The Stationery Office.

Royal College of Nursing (2003) A Framework for Adult Cancer Nursing. London: RCN Publications.

Thomas K (2003) The Gold Standards Framework in community palliative care. European
    Journal of Palliative Care 10: 113-15

Woodman CB, Gibbs A, Scott N et al. (2001) Are differences in stage at presentation a
    credible explanation for reported differences in the survival of patients with colorectal
    cancer in Europe? British Journal of Cancer 85: 787-90.

World Health Organization, International Agency for Research on Cancer and European
    Commission (1995) Survival of Cancer Patients in Europe: The Eurocare study. Lyon:
    IARC Scientific Publications, No. 132.

Part 1
The nature of bowel cancer

Chapter 1

The biological basis of bowel cancer

Barry Rawlings

Cancer is not a new disease. It is often thought of as a twentieth-century phenomenon, but archaeological records show that cancer was known to the ancient Egyptians. We, however, live to an age at which cancer is more likely to affect us, in contrast to our ancestors, for whom infection and trauma were common harbingers of morbidity and mortality. Most people, by succumbing to such disasters, did not live long enough to experience cancer.

This chapter, while attempting to clarify the nature of cancer in general terms, focuses mainly on the disease as it involves the bowel.

Terminology

Neoplasm

This refers simply to an abnormal 'new growth' (literal translation) or tumour, benign or malignant.

Tumour

This refers to a solid swelling; originally, it meant any swelling, including that caused by oedema. So a tumour can also be called a neoplasm, if the latter is used in its literal sense.

Benign tumour

This has well-defined margins, with local growth but no spread. Microscope examination shows the cells resembling almost exactly the cells from which they derive, and so such a growth is referred to as being 'differentiated'. As they resemble their origins, i.e. being differentiated, benign tumour cells often continue to perform the function of the tissue of origin.

Malignant tumour

This has poorly defined margins, with invasion of surrounding tissue. Its cells can differ from those of the tissue of origin to a lesser or greater extent:

- Well-differentiated tumour: cells retain a close resemblance to the original tissue
- Poorly differentiated tumour: cells have little resemblance to their origins
- Anaplastic tumour: cells have totally lost their original characteristics.

In the last example, it is impossible to tell from which tissue the growth came and such malignancies usually offer a poor prognosis. Generally, the poorer the degree of differentiation in a malignant tumour the more aggressive is its behaviour in terms of invasion and spread, and so, generally, the less favourable the prognosis (Stevens and Lowe 2000).

Various abnormalities can occur in malignant tissue and within individual malignant cells; these abnormal features become more obvious with increasing loss of differentiation. There is, of course, an increase in cell numbers which reflects an increase in mitotic activity and, consequently, excessive cell division. Organs that normally have a rapid rate of cell division and turnover are not necessarily associated with an increased risk of malignancy. The small bowel, for example, is such an organ, yet malignant tumours are rarely found there. So, clearly, there have to be other characteristics in order that we can state that malignancy is present. Examples of such other features (Figure 1.1) may include (Franks 1997, Stevens and Lowe 2000):

- Loss of the normal arrangement of cells
- Variation in the shape and size of cells
- Increase in the variation in the shape and size of nuclei
- Increase in the size of nuclei relative to the size of the cytoplasm
- Increased density of staining in the nuclei
- Abnormal mitoses and abnormal chromosomes.

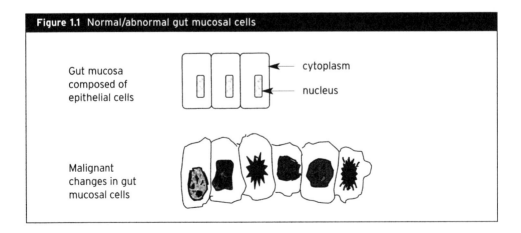

Figure 1.1 Normal/abnormal gut mucosal cells

Gut mucosa composed of epithelial cells — cytoplasm, nucleus

Malignant changes in gut mucosal cells

Dysplasia

Cells show some features that are usually associated with malignant cells. Examples of such features are:

- An increase in mitosis rate
- Incomplete maturation, e.g. nuclei are irregular, large.

Dysplasia is not a malignant situation in itself but malignant change may follow in time. An example is colonic mucosa, in some patients with ulcerative colitis of a long-standing nature, undergoing progression from dysplasia to neoplasia.

A stage called neoplasia *in situ* (carcinoma *in situ*) is often seen in epithelial cells before full malignancy where no invasion of local tissue has yet occurred (Stevens and Lowe 2000).

So what of our word 'cancer' with which we started this chapter? In some ways, it is a helpful term. It suggests the image of a crab using its claws to take hold of the surrounding material – a reasonable image when considering the invasive nature of a malignant tumour. In other ways, it is a less than helpful word, not least because it fails to distinguish between various types of malignancy. It is often thought, for example, that 'cancer' and 'carcinoma' are one and the same, but the latter term refers only to malignancy arising from epithelial tissue. Bowel 'cancer' is an example of carcinoma because it is in the epithelial lining (the mucosa) of the gut that the malignancy arises. Indeed, as the mucosal epithelium has a glandular-looking structure, and as 'adeno' means glandular, we speak of 'adenocarcinoma' of the bowel. 'Sarcoma' is a malignancy arising from muscle or connective tissue. Yet the word 'cancer' is often used in a blanket fashion to denote either carcinoma or sarcoma. It is, then, a word that lacks specificity. Yet it remains a word that can be used (as in this chapter) if we understand its limitations.

Adenoma

Adenomas can appear in the large intestine, usually as polyps, although some are flat in appearance. A polyp is a mass protruding, in this case, into the lumen of the bowel. Adenomatous polyps are considered to be pre-malignant but the level of risk of a carcinoma developing varies according to the type of polyp (Crawford 1999). This point is explored later. Suffice it to say now that most colorectal carcinomas are thought to arise from pre-existing adenomas, whether polypoid or flat, in the large bowel; not all such adenomas, however, inevitably give rise to carcinomas.

Epidemiology

Colorectal cancer is the second most common cancer affecting both men and women (CCC 2003, National Cancer Guidance Steering Group or NCGSG 2004). It causes around 16 000 deaths per year in the UK with no significant sex difference. Boyle et al. (2000) prefer to consider colonic and rectal cancer as two separate disease entities. They point, for example, to the high rates of colonic carcinoma in a number of African–American populations in the USA, with little difference between the sexes. They also refer to the three- to fourfold increase in risk for offspring of Japanese people who moved to the USA, compared with Japanese remaining in Japan. These authors paint a different picture for rectal cancer, particularly identifying the high rates for both sexes in the Czech Republic and in Japanese population groups both in Japan and in the USA.

Most epidemiological studies refer to the low incidence of colorectal cancer in what are regarded as less developed areas of the world, such as Asia and central Africa.

As with other carcinomas, colorectal cancer occurs mostly in older age groups, with a peak incidence in the UK between 70 and 80 years of age. Over 50% of this type of cancer occurs in individuals who are over 60 years of age; less than 5% of cases are found in the under-40s (Jones 1999). In considering age in bowel cancer, Key et al. (1997) refer to the increased incidence for women between the ages of 25 and 70 in England and Wales during the 1980s. This increase was well over a hundredfold. But when the figures were broken down according to age, it was found that the increase was 0.4 per 100 000 at age 25 and 107.5 per 100 000 at age 70. Since that decade, evidence has been noted of some decrease in incidence in younger age groups (of both sexes) in England and Wales.

The vast majority of cases of colorectal carcinoma, perhaps as many as 90% (Acheson and Scholefield 2002), are sporadic. In such cases, there is no evidence of hereditary syndromes such as familial adenomatous polyposis (FAP) or hereditary non-polyposis colorectal cancer (HNPCC). Both syndromes, described later, together account for under 10% of colorectal cancers. In sporadic cases, there is no past or current disease, such as long-standing ulcerative colitis, that may predispose the patient to developing colorectal cancer. Bateman (2003) suggests, however, that about 25% of sporadic bowel cancers may show familial clustering, in that the malignancy is seen in more than one family member but with no obvious inheritance pattern.

In summary, colorectal carcinoma is a disease that, for both sexes of middle age and older, features high in the 'league table' of cancers seen in the UK. It is also clear that most cases cannot be predicted from heredity patterns.

Aetiology

A minority of cases of colorectal carcinoma arise from inherited specific genetic defects, as mentioned above; these defects are found in sex cells, hence their high risk of transmissibility to affected people's offspring. The great majority of bowel cancer cases, however, are not inherited in those ways and so arise from alterations, not in sex cells, but in body (somatic) cells. This section focuses on environmental factors that are suspected of having a role in the genetic (but non-inherited) changes that occur in somatic cells, and therefore are implicated in the causes of sporadic colorectal cancer.

The role of environmental factors must not be underestimated. In considering epidemiology above, it was seen that the incidence of colon cancer among Japanese individuals varied between migrants' offspring in the USA and residents of Japan. The conclusion is that the occurrence of the disease is related to environmental factors that differ in the two countries.

Some of the factors that may play a part in colorectal cancer feature in aetiological lists for other malignancies. Diet, cigarette smoking and alcohol consumption are prime examples. This is not to argue that factors such as radiation and the so-called oncogenic viruses, which feature in lists of general causes of cancer, have no role in colorectal malignancy. We briefly consider these two factors before a more detailed analysis of the factors more commonly associated with this cancer.

The increase in colon cancer seen among the survivors of the atomic bombs in Hiroshima and Nagasaki (Cotran et al. 1999) is often overlooked. Attention usually focuses on the marked increase in certain forms of leukaemia that occurred in those cities over the following few years; solid tumours, such as colon carcinoma with its relatively long latent period, did not appear until some time later. It should be said, however, that, aside from such extreme examples as atomic energy, radiation-induced malignancy in the gastrointestinal tract is unusual. But, as Cotran et al. (1999) remind us, sufficient doses of radiation can change any body cell into a malignant one.

Oncogenic viruses are those viruses that are associated with cancer development. Although there is no evidence for such a type of virus playing any role in colorectal cancer, it is perhaps worth pointing out that DNA of a particular human papillomavirus (HPV) – subtype HPV 16 – is commonly found in a number of carcinomas, including that of the anus (Baumforth et al. 2001).

Dietary factors

Cummings and Bingham (1998) point to assertions that diet may account for up to 80% of large bowel cancers. It is certainly logical to look for an association between this type of malignancy and what we eat. It is not necessarily always the case that what we actually eat is carcinogenic. As Jones (1999) reminds us, some of the foodstuffs we ingest may be rendered carcinogenic only when they undergo chemical change in the gastrointestinal tract. It is also some food preservatives, not just the food itself, that may be rendered carcinogenic, e.g. nitrate-containing preservative is converted to carcinogens by the gut flora (the normal bacterial inhabitants of the human gut).

It is generally believed by most workers in the field that red meat and animal fat are probable risk factors, as are low intakes of fibre and vegetables. 'Red meat' includes beef, pork and lamb. Cummings and Bingham (1998) refer to two studies of health professionals in the USA, where it was concluded that two portions of red meat daily gave the highest relative risk of bowel cancer, whereas two portions of red meat weekly offered the least risk. Also implicated are processed meats, such as sausages, smoked, salted or cured meat, and canned meat.

Meat may increase colorectal cancer risk in several ways, e.g. it is thought that high red meat or low fibre intake can increase levels of ammonia and other nitrogen-containing compounds in the faeces, and that these compounds may be carcinogenic (Key et al. 1997). Substances known as heterocyclic amines (derivatives of ammonia) are formed on the surface of meat when it is roasted, grilled, fried or barbecued. Some people have a liver enzyme system less well equipped than others to safely metabolize these amines; such individuals have a higher risk of adenoma formation and bowel cancer (Cummings and Bingham 1998). Animal fat, eaten as part of meat or in other forms, is thought to lead to increased synthesis of bile acids which can act as carcinogenic agents, either directly or following breakdown by the gut flora.

Dietary fibre, or non-starch polysaccharide to give it its correct name, is thought to reduce colorectal cancer risk in multiple ways. Its ability to reduce the time faeces stay in the gut lumen by encouraging regular defecation clearly also reduces the time for carcinogenic substances to act adversely on bowel mucosa. Fibre also may bind to carcinogens, be they bile acids, ammonia or other nitrogenous compounds, thus reducing their levels in the gut (Key et al. 1997). Fibre may do even more. Its fermentation in the large bowel leads to the formation of substances that may offer protection by stopping excess cell growth and causing cells that have damaged DNA (a potential cancer risk) to undergo a carefully regulated and physiologically normal form of cell death, known as apoptosis (Cummings and Bingham 1998).

There have been suggestions that the presence of free radicals can increase the risk of bowel cancer. These ideas have led to some workers looking at the roles of antioxidants, such as vitamins A, C and E, in the diet. Definitive proof is still awaited, and all are agreed that vitamin supplements are to be avoided because they may be harmful in other ways.

Cigarette smoking and alcohol consumption

Regular intake of cigarette smoke of any amount probably constitutes a risk for developing colorectal carcinoma, whereas only a fairly high intake of alcohol on a regular basis is likely to be problematic. Qualifying comments need to be made here. As Brown and Bishop (2000) point out, studies of smoking have shown a positive association with bowel cancer risk, but it is a weak one. Also, it is possible that alcohol may be more of a risk factor for rectal carcinoma than it is for colon malignancy. Salaspuro (2003), however, questions the dose-dependent approach in relation to alcohol being a risk factor for bowel cancer, citing evidence that moderate or even low alcohol intake can lead to an increased risk. A substance called acetaldehyde is produced from alcohol in the breakdown of the latter, and it is suspected by some that acetaldehyde may be carcinogenic to the large bowel.

Other factors

It is interesting to note that insufficient physical activity has been explored as a risk factor for various malignancies. There is evidence that physical activity offers a protective influence against colonic, but not rectal, cancer. Apart from the resulting positive effect of frequent, regular defecation, with consequent reduced time for exposure of gut mucosa to carcinogens, physical activity may have beneficial effects on substances, including bile acids, that influence colonic cell growth and division (Batty and Thune 2000).

As indicated in the section on epidemiology, there is a subset of patients for whom the main aetiological driving force for their colorectal cancer is inflammatory bowel disease. The main risk seems to apply to ulcerative colitis sufferers who have had the disease for more than 10 years and who have the inflammatory process active in at least the whole of the left colon and rectum (Acheson and Scholefield 2002). Patients with Crohn's disease in the colon also have an increased risk of cancer, but the risk is less than for colitis sufferers.

It should be added that individuals who have had colorectal carcinoma previously have an increased risk of developing a further such cancer.

Finally, as already indicated, some kinds of bowel polyp may confer an increased risk of colorectal cancer, because such adenomatous tumours are considered to be pre-malignant. Table 1.1 summarizes the aetiology and risk factors of colorectal carcinoma.

Table 1.1 Aetiology and high-risk factors in colorectal carcinoma	
Genetic	FAP: HNPCC
Inflammatory bowel disease	Especially ulcerative colitis
Environmental	Dietary factors Cigarette smoking Alcohol intake, especially for rectal carcinoma Physical activity (Radiation) (Oncogenic viruses)
Certain types of bowel adenoma	
Previous colorectal carcinoma	

Pathology I: carcinogenesis

Having defined some terms, and considered the incidence and possible causes of colorectal carcinoma, we now explore how this cancer develops. Much of what follows applies to the development of cancers in general. Carcinogenesis, i.e. the formation and development of cancer, is thought to comprise certain stages.

Initiation stage

This stage renders cells susceptible to becoming malignant should they meet promoting agents (see below). It occurs as a result of exposure to a carcinogen known as an initiating agent, which brings about change (mutation) in certain genes in the affected cells. That change may persist for a long time, perhaps even years. It is commonly supposed that one cell is altered in this way and that the growth of the cancer arises from proliferation of that changed cell. Yet, it may not be the case that malignant tumours arise from a single cell (Franks 1997). Whatever the truth of this debate, the initiation stage is essential for cancer to develop at a later stage.

Promotion stage

Carcinogens called promoting agents stimulate the initiated cell or cells to divide in an uncontrolled way. It is thought that only prolonged, not transient, exposure of initiated cells to promoters enables onset of the subsequent progression stage. This may explain why some pre-malignant cells do not develop beyond a certain stage, although, as Franks (1997) reminds us, interrupted development could also suggest that there must be growth-inhibiting factors that can counteract the action of promoting carcinogens.

Progression stage

If cell proliferation persists, initiated cells undergo further gene alterations, leading to continuing uncontrolled cell division, producing dysplastic cells, and, ultimately, the development of an invasive malignant growth.

In terms of sporadic colorectal carcinoma, we see a sequence of events, involving a multistage process, which is referred to as the 'adenoma–carcinoma sequence' and explored below. Before giving attention to gene changes, further mention must be made of carcinogens. Tennant et al. (1997) suggest that there are two groups of carcinogens:

- Complete: can produce malignant change on their own
- Incomplete: require promoting agents after initiation occurs, so they cannot produce malignancy on their own.

Promoting agents are not carcinogenic in themselves, because they promote malignancy only after initiation, although they may cause tumour development in cases where there was previous exposure to a 'subthreshold dose' (Tennant et al. 1997, p. 113) of a complete carcinogen. Such a low dose would not itself lead to malignant change.

So complete carcinogens, unlike incomplete ones, can be both initiators and promoters (assuming a 'full' dose). To complicate the picture further, it is thought that some substances can be complete carcinogens in one tissue and incomplete in another.

We must now consider the gene alterations brought about by carcinogens. So that the stages of carcinogenesis can proceed as outlined above, a number of genetic mechanisms can play a role. Two important examples of relevant gene types are given here:

1. Tumour-suppressor genes, the protein products of which normally regulate cell growth by inhibitory influences, become inactive and so allow tumour cells to develop
2. Proto-oncogenes, the protein products of which normally stimulate normal cell growth and differentiation, are transformed into oncogenes (cancer-causing genes), the protein products of which are abnormal and so stimulate inappropriate cell growth.

In sporadic colorectal carcinoma, the so-called 'adenoma–carcinoma sequence' relates to a sequence of gene alterations (Brown and Bishop 2000), most of which involve loss of gene material or gene activation.

The first alteration or mutation, occurring in up to 80% of sporadic cases, is in the *APC* or adenomatous polyposis coli gene, located on the long arm of chromosome 5. The *APC* gene is a tumour-suppressor gene and so its loss of activity leads to gut mucosal cell proliferation and adenoma formation.

An oncogene known as k-*ras*, located on the short arm of chromosome 12, is activated in the polyp cells in about 50% of sporadic cases, resulting in further abnormal growth of tumour cells.

Then a gene called the deletion in colon carcinoma, or *DCC*, gene undergoes mutation. *DCC*, located on the long arm of chromosome 18, is thought to be an example of a tumour-suppressor gene, but doubt has been raised about this belief; there is probably some other gene close to *DCC*'s position on chromosome 18 that is responsible for progression of the malignancy-forming sequence (Cotran et al. 1999).

The last mutation occurring in 70–80% of the sporadic cases occurs in a tumour-suppressor gene, located on the short arm of chromosome 17, known as *p53*, the mutation occurring around the time of the adenomatous cells becoming malignant. This gene undergoes mutation in many types of cancers; *p53* normally brings about apoptosis (defined earlier) of cells with genetic damage. Some workers believe that an altered *p53* gene may allow cancer cells that metastasize, i.e. spread, to other body regions to survive in those novel surroundings (Brown and Bishop 2000).

There are other gene mutations involved in colorectal carcinoma, some of which are not fully understood as yet.

Pathology II: adenoma–carcinoma sequence

As said earlier, most bowel cancers arise from pre-existing adenomas; the phrase 'adenoma–carcinoma sequence' describes this idea (Figure 1.2). Hermanek (2000) refers to a 'dysplasia–carcinoma sequence' when he points out that this phrase covers the pathological mechanism for all colorectal cancer presentations, including cases arising from inflammatory bowel disease. Most workers continue to use the older term.

Bateman (2003) points out that, although adenomas usually occur as polyps, some may be flat in appearance. Those that are polypoid may have a stalk or be sessile (broad based). Their microscopic structure may be tubular (gland-like) or, rarely in the colon, villous (with finger-like projections). Rectal adenomas are usually sessile and villous in type. Colon

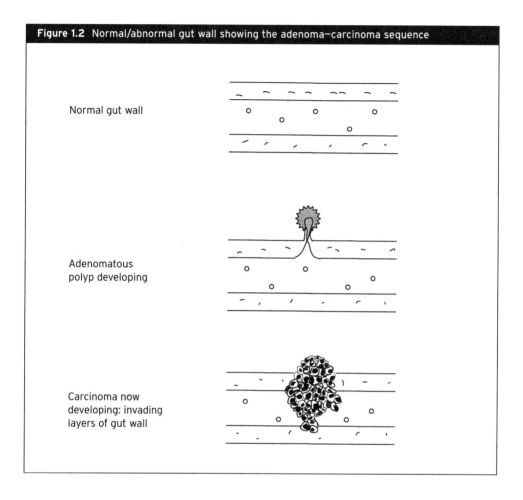

Figure 1.2 Normal/abnormal gut wall showing the adenoma–carcinoma sequence

Normal gut wall

Adenomatous
polyp developing

Carcinoma now
developing: invading
layers of gut wall

adenomas may be mixed in histology (tubulovillous). Large bowel polyps can occur in which there is no malignant tendency. Hence, it is important to focus on adenomas that have the potential to become malignant over a 10- to 15-year period. Yet not all such adenomas give rise to malignancy. Acheson and Scholefield (2002) state that adenomas are considered to be 'high risk' for malignancy when:

- more than two are present
- they are large (1–2 cm or more)
- they are flat, sessile or villous
- their cells display high-grade dysplasia.

Before going on to consider sporadic colorectal carcinoma further, mention must be made of the two hereditary conditions referred to earlier.

Familial adenomatous polyposis

Accounting for less than 1% of colorectal cancers, this condition involves a mutation of the *APC* gene which, as this is an autosomal dominant disease, has a 50:50 chance of being transmitted by an affected parent to an offspring. At least 100 polyps will be present throughout the large bowel; usually far more (up to 2000 or so) are found, and some may be seen in other parts of the gastrointestinal tract. It is likely that FAP has a frequency of progression to bowel malignancy of close to 100% (Crawford 1999), some patients being under 40 when presenting with cancerous changes.

Hereditary non-polyposis colorectal cancer

Accounting for 5% or so of colorectal cancers, HNPCC is an autosomal dominant disease involving mutation of a number of genes (*hMSH2, hMLH1, hPMS1, hPMS2*, found on various chromosomes) responsible for repairing DNA defects. Often a right-sided colon cancer, it usually presents before the age of 50 years and can involve multiple bowel cancers and malignancy in other sites, e.g. endometrium. As Brown and Bishop (2000) point out, polyps not being a prominent feature, there is no obvious clinical marker and so family history of early onset bowel cancer with an autosomal dominant pattern is an indicator.

Pathology III: course of disease

Sporadic colorectal adenocarcinoma is the focus for this final section in the chapter. The distribution of these cancers is as follows (Figure 1.3):

- Up to about 60% in rectosigmoid area
- 20-25% in caecum or ascending colon
- Remainder in transverse or descending colons.

The developing tumour evolves into one of several possible forms, e.g. it may take a ring-like form (annular) which often causes obstructive symptoms by its encircling mode of growth in the bowel wall. The tumour may have an ulcerated appearance and bleed easily. Some tumours retain the appearance of their polypoid origins (Mortensen 2000). The last are found mainly in the caecum and ascending colon; the other two usually occur more distally.

As with any cancer, there is apoptosis of tumour cells as well as rapid cell division but, in colorectal cancer, the latter exceeds the former by only

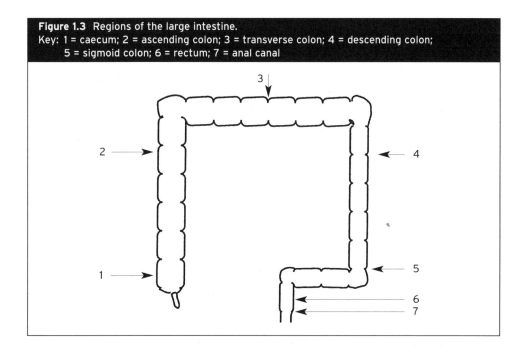

Figure 1.3 Regions of the large intestine.
Key: 1 = caecum; 2 = ascending colon; 3 = transverse colon; 4 = descending colon;
5 = sigmoid colon; 6 = rectum; 7 = anal canal

about 10% and so the carcinoma grows slowly; after clinical diagnosis, a colon cancer doubles its size in 2–3 months (Cotran et al. 1999).

An important factor in influencing malignant cell growth is tumour angiogenesis (Stevens and Lowe 2000). In order to grow, the malignancy requires an adequate blood supply. Diffusion of nutrients and oxygen from existing blood vessels becomes insufficient once the tumour exceeds about 2 mm in diameter. A number of chemicals are secreted by both the tumour cells and inflammatory cells (invariably found within a malignancy); these chemicals stimulate new blood vessels to bud from existing ones and penetrate the tumour, thus directly bringing it nutrients and oxygen. Interestingly, malignant, and other, cells can produce chemicals that prevent or reduce angiogenesis. (A future therapy may lie here, if those 'anti-angiogenic' substances can be harnessed.) Angiogenesis is essential not only for tumour growth, but also for its invasion and metastatic spread.

Invasion and metastasis

As with any carcinoma, growth occurs into adjacent tissue, destroying it. This process of invasion may not occur quickly in colorectal cancer because it can be slow growing; in rectal tumours, it may be 18 months from the beginning of neoplasia until the perirectal tissue is invaded (Williams 2000).

In order to invade, tumour cells must breach the basement membrane, a thin layer found next to the base of the epithelial cells that make up the mucosa. This action is facilitated by reducing some chemicals (e.g. cadherins) that normally cause cells to adhere to each other. Thus, some cancer cells can break away from the primary tumour and move through the basement membrane and matrix of connective tissue that separate them from nearby lymphatic and blood vessels. The malignant cells' journey is aided by their production of enzymes (e.g. proteases) that break down basement membrane and matrix components. Increased motility of the tumour cells also occurs, possibly because they produce chemical motility factors (Stevens and Lowe 2000).

When they reach the lymphatic and blood circulations, these 'breakaway' cancer cells adhere to each other and to blood cells such as platelets. This aggregation increases both the survival of cancer cells in circulation and, later, their ability to leave vessels where the latter are supplying distant organs. It is probable, however, that many tumour cells fail to metastasize as a result of their destruction by immune cells while still in circulation (Cotran et al. 1999).

The most common site for metastases ('secondaries') in colorectal carcinoma is the liver; the lungs are the second most common, with other organs being possible, although less common, sites. Lymphatic spread is probably the most common route of metastasis, but blood-borne spread is also important, e.g. in creating liver metastases. Another method of metastasis that may occur is by some cancer cells, which have penetrated the bowel wall, escaping into the peritoneal cavity and seeding on to lower organs (transcoelomic spread). Mechanisms by which tumour cells metastasize, i.e. enter, and seed in, an organ, are not fully understood, although metastases appear to undergo secondary angiogenesis.

The signs and symptoms of colorectal carcinoma are explored in Chapter 3. Here it suffices to summarize the local and systemic effects of this cancer in Table 1.2.

Summary of key points

- Colorectal carcinoma features high in the 'league table' of malignancy in the UK.
- Most cases are sporadic, with no obvious hereditary pattern; less than 10% of cases have a well-recognized pattern of inheritance.
- Several causative influences are thought likely in colorectal cancer, dietary factors being considered particularly important.
- The stages of development and gene changes of colorectal cancer are well documented.

Table 1.2 Some effects of colorectal carcinoma

Local

- Invasion
- Pressure on adjacent structures
- Impairment/loss of function
- Bowel obstruction
- Intussusception (infrequent)
- Ulceration, through adjacent structures
- Bleeding

Systemic

- Metastasis
- Cachexia (wasting), from cytokine* secretion by cancer cells or macrophages
- Clotting imbalance:
  - → venous thrombosis
  - → disseminated intravascular coagulation
- Anaemia from bleeding, cachexia or marrow infiltration by cancer cells or their products

* Chemical mediators, normally produced by immune cells with a variety of actions.

References

Acheson AG, Scholefield JH (2002) What is new in colorectal cancer? Surgery 20(10): 244-8.

Bateman AC (2003) Pathology of small and large intestinal tumours. Surgery 21(2): iii-vi.

Batty D, Thune I (2000) Does physical activity prevent cancer? British Medical Journal 321: 424-5.

Baumforth K, Murray PG, Young LS (2001) Tumour viruses and human cancer. In: Phillips J, Murray P, Kirk P (eds), The Biology of Disease, 2nd edn. Oxford: Blackwell Science, pp. 204-13.

Boyle P, Burns HJG, Gray N et al. (2000) Epidemiology of colorectal cancer control. In: McArdle CS, Kerr DJ, Boyle P (eds), Colorectal Cancer. Oxford: Isis Medical Media, pp. 1-31.

Brown SR, Bishop DT (2000) Genetics of colorectal cancer. In: McArdle CS, Kerr DJ, Boyle P (eds), Colorectal Cancer. Oxford: Isis Medical Media, pp. 71-86.

Colon Cancer Concern (2003) Viewpoint: Colon Cancer Roadshow. Cancer Nursing Practice 2: 16-17.

Cotran RS, Kumar V, Collins T (1999) Robbins Pathologic Basis of Disease, 6th edn. Philadelphia: WB Saunders.

Crawford JM (1999) The gastrointestinal tract. In: Cotran RS, Kumar V, Collins T (eds), Robbins Pathologic Basis of Disease, 6th edn. Philadelphia: WB Saunders, pp. 775-844.

Cummings JH, Bingham SA (1998) Diet and the prevention of cancer. British Medical Journal 317: 1636-40.

Franks LM (1997) What is cancer? In: Franks LM, Teich NM (eds), Introduction to the Cellular and Molecular Biology of Cancer, 3rd edn. Oxford: Oxford University Press, pp. 1-20.

Hermanek P (2000) Pathology of colorectal cancer and premalignant lesions. In: McArdle CS, Kerr DJ, Boyle P (eds), Colorectal Cancer. Oxford: Isis Medical Media, pp. 57-70.

Jones DJ (1999) Colorectal neoplasia - II: large bowel cancer. In: Jones DJ (ed.), ABC of Colorectal Diseases, 2nd edn. London: BMJ Books, pp. 64-7.

Key T, Forman D, Pike MC (1997) Epidemiology of cancer. In: Franks LM, Teich NM (eds), Introduction to the Cellular and Molecular Biology of Cancer, 3rd edn. Oxford: Oxford University Press, pp. 34–59.

Mortensen NJMcC (2000) The small and large intestines. In: Russell RCG, Williams NS, Bulstrode CJK (eds), Bailey and Love's Short Practice of Surgery, 23rd edn. London: Arnold, pp. 1026–57.

National Cancer Guidance Steering Group (2004) Improving Outcomes in Colorectal Cancer. Manual update. London: NICE.

Salaspuro MP (2003) Alcohol consumption and cancer of the gastrointestinal tract. In: Tytgat G NJ (ed.), Best Practice and Research: Clinical gastroenterology. London: Baillière Tindall, pp. 679–94.

Stevens A, Lowe J (2000) Pathology, 2nd edn. Edinburgh: Mosby.

Tennant R, Wigley C, Balmain A (1997) Chemical carcinogenesis. In: Franks LM, Teich NM (eds), Introduction to the Cellular and Molecular Biology of Cancer, 3rd edn. Oxford: Oxford University Press, pp. 106–29.

Williams NS (2000) The rectum. In: Russell RCG, Williams NS, Bulstrode CJK (eds), Bailey and Love's Short Practice of Surgery, 23rd edn. London: Arnold, pp. 1093–114.

Further reading

Flower R (2003) What are all the things aspirin does? (Editorial). British Medical Journal 327: 572–3.

Phillips J, Murray P, Kirk P (eds) (2001) The Biology of Disease, 2nd edn. Oxford: Blackwell Science, Chapters 21, 22, 23 and 24.

Chapter 2

Prevention, screening and early detection

Barbara Borwell

Many of the cancers affecting society today can be cured if detected early; not only are some of these curable, they are also preventable. Colorectal cancer (CRC) is among those malignancies that may be controlled through early detection, and the key to prevention is education in healthy practices, plus the vigilance of doctors and health-care workers.

This chapter briefly explores the rationale for promoting a positive approach to health and discusses opportunities, and activities, that can influence bowel cancer prevention.

There is now substantial evidence to suggest that deaths from bowel cancer could be prevented by earlier detection and diagnosis. Political and social forces influence health promotion activities, but most health-care workers accept that some kind of prioritization in health care is essential. Improvement in the survival rate from bowel cancer with educational and health protection activities, founded on current national and local initiatives, acknowledges the contribution of doctors and health-care workers in their goal to improve the nation's survival rate from bowel cancer.

It is beyond the scope of this chapter to provide a comprehensive account of health promotion; literature is widely available on the topic. The concept of health is explored to offer clarity for the reader.

What is health?

Attempts to define the meaning of health, it could be argued, have stemmed from the World Health Organization's original and classic definition of health (WHO, 1946) where it advocated a positive and holistic state of health and well-being, physically, mentally and socially, and not merely disease prevention and control. This could be viewed as having negative and positive connotations – negative because it does not infer disease or disability, positive with inference being on a quality status. An individual's perception of health will differ from individual to individual, and it is essential that health promoters understand their own concept of health as well as the values held by their clients. Effectual communication about health issues is reliant on this understanding. WHO (1984) further expanded and clarified the concept and principles of health, health in this context now being seen as an essential and complex resource and aid to daily living, not the sole purpose for living. This takes into account physical abilities, and personal and social circumstances. It is what enables the individual to adapt, change and cope in a constantly changing world.

Health promotion

Health is fundamental to our existence and health promotion must assist people to attain enhanced health rather than seek to reach a specified stage of health, thus increasing the overall capacity of better health for individuals and communities. Health promoters and agencies must therefore seek to prevent ill-health, and at the same time consider ways to improve and enable positive health, mindful of their potential contributions. Individually, goals may not be attainable collectively; the optimum is more likely to be achieved. Educating for health is concerned with influencing beliefs, attitudes and behaviour of the determinants of health, including those with power and the community at large (WHO 1978). The basic principle of health education and health promotion is empowerment, helping people to take greater control of their lives. Promotion and support of a healthier lifestyle that involves personal, social and environmental changes require the development of strategies and partnerships between organizations and the target population.

Lifestyle beliefs and behaviours in relation to health are not without their own controversies. The concept of lifestyle can be used by professionals as an interventionist approach to legitimize disease-related activities and evade the social responsibility for ill-health, rather than focus on the equities and disparities that characterize the population as a whole. Policy-makers can also use this approach as an excuse to evade responsibility for the social causes of ill-health (Gott and O'Brien 1990). Within the past decade health promotion has received much publicity and government investment in the UK. The launch of England's *The Health of the Nation Strategy* (Department of Health or DoH 1992) happened, in which, in collaboration with statutory and voluntary organizations and involvement of local communities, strategies and priorities for health improvement have been established to address key issues. In Scotland, Wales and Northern Ireland similar strategies and policies have been implemented to improve health in areas of concern (Health Promotion

Authority for Wales 1990, Northern Ireland Department of Health and Social Security or NIDHSS 1991, Scottish Office Home and Health Department or SOHHD 1991, Scottish Office 1992). All of these strategies have provided significant opportunities for developing healthy alliances and initiatives with organizations to improve the nation's health.

Based on this idea of 'doing', Tannahill (1985), cited in Downie et al. (1996), developed a model to support those concerned in health promotion to define and plan their interventions (Figure 2.1). This model signifies the overlap of health education, prevention and health protection, and interdependence, suggesting that effective health promotion strategies require collaborative action between interdisciplinary healthcare workers:

- Health education (the doing part of health promotion), e.g. development and training in life skills, empowering and helping people to have control of their lives.
- Prevention: identifying and implementing services that seek to prevent ill-health and disease, e.g. bowel cancer awareness and screening.
- Health protection: establishing national and local strategies legislation aimed at protecting the community from social behaviours known to cause harm, e.g. to deter drug abuse.

Figure 2.1 A model of health promotion. (From Tannahill 1985, adapted from Downie et al. 1996, Figure 4.1, p. 59. By permission of Oxford University Press.)

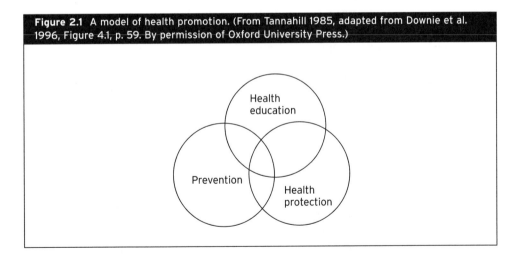

Spheres of overlap

- Preventive health education: includes information, communication and the identification of those individuals in the population most vulnerable and known to be at higher risk.

- Preventive health protection: examples include control of crop spraying with those pesticides known to have links to cancer and other conditions.
- Health education aimed at health protection: adopting a proactive stance with policy makers and the community about why certain actions are desirable through commitment, communication, education and appropriate research.

Preventive health education and planning for prevention

Health education is about messages and activity aimed at improving or maximizing health and preventing or reducing ill-health, through communication to individuals or groups. Bowel cancer can, for some, cause embarrassment and is not a topic that people generally want to talk about. The cultural perception of cancer is imbued with particular meaning and evokes a unique fear, representing a skewed body perception and a feeling of helplessness.

Downie et al. (1996) imply that the community response to health promotion initiatives is connected to health-related beliefs and behaviour; consequently attitudes are frequently perceived to be central to health promotion. Development of effective health promotion programmes requires those actively engaged to have an understanding of attitudes within a specific viewpoint and of the interrelationship of environmental circumstances, individual characteristics, culture and society.

Reduction in the incidence and mortality rate of bowel cancer requires change in public beliefs and attitude about the disease. Long-term commitment relies on raising public awareness, and encouraging understanding of and openness about risk factors associated with bowel cancer. Health educators can adopt an ethical stance to facilitate and generate understanding through empowerment, translating reliable knowledge and information for individuals and the wider community.

This approach is compatible with Becker's (1974) 'health belief model' in supporting cancer screening programme activities. The concept of the model is based on individuals' perception of their risks of developing bowel cancer, leading to preventive strategies being noticeably beneficial.

A family diagnosis of bowel cancer frequently increases concern about individual vulnerability to the disease; this is not necessarily reflected in other conditions where there is awareness associated with certain types of behaviour but not perceived risk. Beliefs therefore differ about the positive and negative effects of establishing a behaviour change.

Cancer is widely associated with a significant death risk and with a serious diagnosis, suggesting that individual lifestyle and behaviour changes are more likely to be effective, although not necessarily easily achieved.

Effective health education relies on good communication when planning activity to improve health, thereby reducing the risk of ill-health. Helping people to understand the costs, benefits and process of change requires a programme that is flexible, transferable and respectful of individuals or communities. The change process for some can be destabilizing; feelings of inadequacy may be displayed, regressing to the phase of thinking about change. Support, reassurance and possibly further education are needed to reinforce that the programme can be re-joined at any time.

The community development model (Heller et al. 1989) is attuned with this plan, relying on unity between health workers and organizations from programme inception through to delivery and evaluation.

Screening and early detection

Two different types of screening are described: opportunistic and population based.

Opportunistic screening is when a person makes a decision to seek advice to confirm his or her health, such as well-woman clinics where specific routine tests are performed that pertain to frequently occurring conditions.

Population screening targets a healthy population who fulfil specified criteria and attend by invitation to exclude certain diseases.

The incidence of CRC in both developed and developing countries is increasing and frequently associated with diet and lifestyle. The American Cancer Society (ACS) estimate that about 129 400 new cases of CRC were diagnosed in 1999, claiming approximately 58 000 lives; it is the second leading cause of death in the USA (American Cancer Society 1999). An estimated 33 000 new cases of CRC are diagnosed annually in the UK, accounting for some 16 000 deaths (Colon Cancer Concern 2003). Overall the 5-year survival rate is around 45%, acknowledging regional variations (National Cancer Guidance Steering Group or NCGSG 2004); after curative surgery this can reach 70%. CRC in its early stages is potentially curable; however, at this stage, symptoms are not usually apparent. Currently, 80% of CRC cases present with advanced disease and poor prognosis.

Primary prevention

Primary prevention activities require a totally asymptomatic population to give specific protection for preventing their occurrence (Pender et al. 2002). Generally, actions related to lifestyle behaviours are considered fundamental.

Diet and lifestyle

Dietary and lifestyle connections are key environmental issues as causative and preventive factors of CRC (Chamberlain 1995, Kim 2000). An estimated 80% of CRCs could be prevented by dietary changes (Cummings and Bingham 1998). In 1969 Burkitt proposed a fibre-rich diet, having noted that the incidence of CRC was lower in African populations compared with western countries, signifying that high-fibre foods are easily digested and add bulk to the stool, so reducing the transit time through the colon. Whittaker (2001), cited in De Snoo (2003, p. 44), noted that 38% of large bowel cancers are in the rectum, thereby supporting Burkitt's (1969) theory; more recently Terry et al. (2001) noted that reducing the stool transit time would decrease the risk of CRC by reducing the contact time between the carcinogenic substances and the rectal mucosa.

Dietary fat is usually a risk factor linked with CRC; however, epidemiological studies suggest that the proportion of fat in the diet is insignificant, the main facts being the entire calorie intake and body mass index (NCGSG 2004). Less established are links between dietary cholesterol and CRC (see also Chapters 1 and 11).

The relationship between consumption of red meat and CRC has also been widely debated, including the working group on diet and cancer of the Committee on Medical Aspects (COMA) (DoH 1997–8). Tuswell's (2002) study failed to establish any connection and the risk difference between vegetarians and control cases was insignificant. The relationship between CRC and certain vitamins requires further evidence.

High levels of alcohol consumption are associated with increased risk of developing adenomas and CRC (DoH 1997–8). Long-term cigarette smoking has recognized connections with chronic disease, including several cancers. Research conducted by Chao et al. (2000) proposes an increased risk of CRC mortality in both men and women. The study reviewed smoking history and number of cigarettes smoked daily/annually, and concluded that current smokers were at most risk; however, the risk reduced after smoking cessation.

Obesity and physical inactivity are other factors linked with an increased risk of CRC development (American Cancer Society 2003, DoH

1997–8). Chapter 1 has more detail on lifestyle and environmental factors associated with CRC.

Chemoprevention or pharmacological prevention is another approach to decrease the mortality rate from CRC, aimed at interfering with the formation of adenomatous polyps and consequential development of CRC (Janne and Mayer 2001).

Chemotherapeutic oral agents known to have this protective effect taken over a long-term period are aspirin and other non-steroidal anti-inflammatory drugs (NSAIDs), folate and calcium supplements and, in postmenopausal women, hormone replacement therapy. Current infrastructure to regulate and evaluate this method within the National Health Service (UK) is an area for future research.

Secondary prevention

Some bowel conditions may increase a person's risk of developing cancer. Earlier detection to reduce morbidity and mortality will be achieved only by screening asymptomatic individuals using safe, reliable diagnostic tests based on recognized guidelines (NHS Centre for Reviews and Dissemination 1997, NCGSG 2004).

Population screening

Screening is not a diagnostic test and not all screening can be seen as beneficial; potential disease could be identified without appropriate measures for the successful treatment of the condition. Confirmation that intervention is beneficial in terms of disease prevention and reducing mortality is a requirement before the implementation of any screening programme.

Before screening can be introduced, the following must be possible:

- The disease must be recognized as a serious health problem. Bowel cancer is the second most common cancer in men and women and the third most common cancer in the UK. Britain's second largest cancer killer claims 16 000 lives each year in the UK (CCC 2003, cited in Viewpoint 2003).
- Its early stages must be detectable. Colorectal cancers are considered to arise from benign polyps, so screening must identify these pre-malignant lesions at an early stage because the prognosis is related to Dukes' staging (see Chapter 3).
- The test must be suitable, reliable, acceptable to the general population and affordable by the public health authority. Current methods are: faecal

occult blood test (FOBT), digital rectal examination (DRE) and flexible
sigmoidoscopy to envisage distal lesions.

- Colonoscopy is primarily a diagnostic tool; however, some genetic
  conditions do have a predisposition to CRC requiring entire colon
  visualization, essentially by colonoscopy

Faecal occult blood test

The FOBT, such as guaiac (Haemoccult), is used to check for non-visible
blood in the stool. This method, developed some 30 years ago, identifies
blood from the colon; blood from other gastrointestinal sources has a
nominal effect (Hart et al. 1995). A small sample of stool is placed on a
guaiac-impregnated card. Three consecutive samples are collected and
then analysed. The test is fairly simple and usually done at home. Diet and
some drugs can generate false positives and influence the results. The positive rate can be reduced by excluding red meat and vegetables that have
a high peroxidase content – namely, cucumber, cauliflower, turnip, grape-
fruit and carrot – from the diet 2 days before the test. Certain drugs can
distort the results, typically aspirin and NSAIDs; these should be avoided.
Vitamin C preparations, which can inhibit peroxidases in haemoglobin,
may produce a false-negative result. Sensitivity of FOBT for unhydration
of the test is between 72 and 78%, with a specificity of 98%. Studies suggest that sensitivity can be increased between 88 and 92% by rehydrating
the slides; however, specificity was decreased to 90% (Hart et al. 1995,
Rawl et al. 2002).

The FOBT is a model for screening; it is safe, non-invasive, easy to use
and inexpensive. The lack of sensitivity to polyps, inability to exclude
everyone from CRC and false positives leading to additional screening
investigations are key considerations. This test meets several screening criteria and improvements are under way to increase diagnostic sensitivity
and specificity. The findings of randomized controlled trials (RCTs) from
the USA, Australia and European countries have shown a 15–33%
decrease in mortality rate using biennial screening on the 50+ age group;
Sweden's final mortality results are pending (Hardcastle et al. 1996,
Kronberg et al. 1996, Towler et al. 1998, Mandel et al. 1999).

Digital rectal examination

This involves examination of the lower rectum. The method is simple and
safe to perform; however, the inserted finger can locate only a small per-
centage of tumours. For population screening its limitations do not fulfil
the criteria.

Flexible sigmoidoscopy

Flexible sigmoidoscopy (sigmoidoscopy) is an invasive procedure that can visualize the lower half of the colon up to the splenic flexure. This procedure is more sensitive than FOBT for detecting distal tumours and polyps. This investigation relies on the skill of the individual performing the examination, especially the depth of insertion of the scope. Sigmoidoscopy has been estimated to identify 65% of all patients with significant colonic lesions, but can identify only lesions in the rectum or about 60 cm distally (Midgley and Kerr 1999, p. 394). Detection of abnormalities by sigmoidoscope automatically indicates further investigations to examine the entire colon. The false-positive rate by endoscopic screening is difficult to quantify; many low, potentially malignant polyps may be removed through screening, placing these people into long-term surveillance programmes.

Colonoscopy

Colonoscopy allows visualization of the entire colon. Reports have aroused discussion about the feasibility of colonoscopy as a screening test, either at 10-year intervals or as a once in a lifetime procedure for people aged between 55 and 65. The probability of its use as a screening tool for CRC is debatable, in spite of predictions that the mortality rate could be reduced by 70% (Midgley and Kerr 1999). It is expensive, with sigmoidoscopy being seen as a 'second best' approach.

Based on the natural history of the disease, CRC is ideally suited to screening (see Chapter 1). Identification of an abnormal result may highlight a person's risk from the disease, requiring further investigations. Early detection, when the disease is potentially curable, is an attractive outlook.

Acceptance of the screening method by the target group and compliance to attain a minimal quota to ensure programme feasibility are essential. Tests that are painless, quick and identify abnormalities, with prompt and successful treatment, are a patient's optimum; in reality, this is not possible. Screening-induced concern has been shown to reflect the type of method used. FOBT, although not an invasive procedure, increased anxiety when the initial result showed false positive, decreasing after medical examination. Further review at 12 months showed that most people were pleased that they had participated (Lindholm et al. 1997). Endoscopy, a more complex procedure, suggests that people are generally receptive to this screening method (Dominitz and Provenzale 1997).

At present, evaluation of the benefits, programme compliance and cost-effectiveness of routine screening of an asymptomatic population in most European countries is not entirely justified. Opinion differs in the USA where screening is well established, based on recommendations from the American Cancer Society:

- DRE annually for people > 40 years
- FOBT annually for people > 50 years
- Sigmoidoscopy 3- to 5-yearly in people > 50 years.

Currently, the UK has no nationwide screening programme for colorectal cancer. In response to the government publication *Improving Outcomes in Colorectal Cancer*, a committee was established to review and evaluate the effectiveness of screening (NHS Executive 1997). The group concluded that substantial evidence warranted UK investigations to reduce the overall mortality rate from CRC (Hardcastle et al. 1996). Recommendations indicated that a pilot study should be established to consider the feasibility and acceptability of the FOBT as a screening tool. The 2-year study aimed at an invited population aged between 50 and 69 years would yield 189 319 individuals in England and 297 036 in Scotland. Areas selected were the west Midlands in England and Tayside, Grampian and Fife in Scotland, seen as representative of the UK population, including ethnic groups, and rural and urban populations. The project was completed in September 2002. The findings conclude that mortality reductions demonstrated from previous randomized studies can be repeated in the screening models used in this study, and recommend that FOBT should become part of a national screening strategy to address CRC (www.cancerscreening.nhs.uk/colorectal/end-of-pilot.html – information last retrieved 25 April 2004).

Evidence from other screening methods such as flexible sigmoidoscopy continues to accumulate. Single-use flexible sigmoidoscopy reviewed on people aged around 60 years reports that the regimen is acceptable, feasible and safe. Baseline findings suggest that the prevalence of neoplasia was important and the availability of a national programme could accomplish similar outcomes to the successful UK breast and cervical cancer screening programmes, provided compliance rates are comparable (Atkin et al. 2002). Focus on how FOBT can best contribute to reduce population mortality from CRC is an important consideration (NHS 2003).

Summary of screening criteria

- Disease must be a significant health problem
- Recognizable early stage disease
- Relevant treatment available

- Early intervention must be of long-term benefit
- Suitable, reliable test
- Acceptability, compliance, feasibility
- Adequate resources to deal with abnormalities
- Outcome must justify costs

Although controversy remains about the appropriateness and preferred method for a national screening programme, there is consensus about the viability and value of screening for people known to be at increased risk of developing the disease. Table 2.1 gives a review of screening methods available.

Table 2.1 Colorectal cancer (CRC) screening: advantages and disadvantages

Advantages	Disadvantages
National screening for CRC	
Early detection would improve survival	Lifestyle disturbance
Digital rectal examination	
Safe, simple to perform	Invasive
	Detects only rectal tumours up to 7 cm
	Not recommended as a screening-alone procedure
Faecal occult blood test	
Non-invasive, fairly simple to perform	Poor compliance
Reasonable cost	Difficult to perform in some patients
	Unpleasant
	Not highly sensitive
	Anxiety provoking
	Detection of blood usually signifies advanced disease
	False-positive rate high
	Significance of population screening not yet determined
Flexible sigmoidoscopy	
Screening and treatment can be concurrent	Generally adenomas do not develop into cancer
> 60% of all CRCs are detectable	Invasive, costly, time-consuming
Precise and highly discriminatory	Sedation needed
Vigilant surveillance could prevent recurrence	Lack of trained endoscopists
Potential reduction in mortality	Bowel preparation needed
	Lifestyle disruption
	May induce false sense of security – not all adenomas detected
	Possible trauma to colon needing hospitalization

High-risk group

Guidelines for CRC screening in high-risk groups have been developed by the British Association of Gastroenterology (BAG) and the Association of Coloproctology for Great Britain and Ireland (ACPGBI) (Table 2.2). Practical differences may occur between countries, although their

Table 2.2 Summary of recommendations for colorectal screening and surveillance in high-risk groups

Disease groups	Screening procedure	Time of initial screen	Screening procedure and interval
Colorectal cancer	Consultation, LFTs and colonoscopy	Colonoscopy within 6 months of resection only if pre-operative colon evaluation incomplete	Liver scan within 2 years postoperatively Colonoscopy 5-yearly until 70 years
Colonic adenomas *Low risk* 1-2 adenomas, both < 1 cm	Colonoscopy	No surveillance or 5 years	Cease follow-up after negative colonoscopy
Intermediate risk 3-4 adenomas, or at least 1 adenoma ≥ 1 cm	Colonoscopy	3 years	Every 3 years until two consecutive negative colonoscopies, then no further surveillance
High risk More than 5 adenomas or ≥ 3 with at least one ≥ 1 cm	Colonoscopy	1 year	Annual colonoscopy until out of this risk group, then interval colonoscopy as per intermediate risk group
Large sessile adenomas removed piecemeal	Colonoscopy or flexible sigmoi-doscopy (depending on polyp location)	3 monthly until no residual colitis 15 years from onset of symptoms	
Ulcerative colitis and Crohn's colitis	Colonoscopy + biopsies every 10 cm	Pancolitis 8 years, left-sided colitis 15 years from onset of symptoms	Colonoscopy 3 yearly in second decade 2 yearly in third decade, subsequently annually
IBD + PSC ± OLT	Colonoscopy	At diagnosis of PSC	Annual colonoscopy with biopsy every 10 cm
Ureterosigmoidostomy	Flexible sig-moidoscopy	10 years after surgery	Flexible sigmoidoscopy annually
Acromegaly	Colonoscopy	At 40 years	Colonoscopy 5 yearly

Table 2.2 Summary of recommendations for colorectal screening and surveillance in high-risk groups contd.

Disease groups	Lifetime risk of death from CRC	Screening procedure	Age at initial screen (years)	Screening procedure and interval
FAP and variants (refer to clinical geneticist)	1 in 2.5	Genetic testing Flexible sig-moidoscopy + OGD	Puberty	Flexible sigmoid-oscopy 12 monthly Colectomy if positive
Juvenile polyposis and Peutz–Jeghers syndrome (refer to clinical geneticist)	1 in 3	Genetic testing Colonoscopy + OGD	Puberty	Flexible sigmoid-oscopy 12 monthly Colectomy if positive
At risk of HNPCC* or more than 2 FDRs (refer to clinical geneti-cist) Also docu-mented MMR gene carriers	1 in 3	Colonoscopy + OGD	Aged 25 or 5 years before earliest CRC in family Gastroscopy age 50 or 5 years before earliest gastric cancer in family	2 yearly colonoscopy and gastroscopy
2 FDRs with colorectal cancer	1 in 6	Colonoscopy	At first consul-tation or at age 35–40 years, whichever is the later	If initial colonoscopy clear then repeat at age 55 years
1 FDR < 45 years with colorectal cancer	1 in 10	Colonoscopy	At first consul-tation or at age 35–40 years whichever is the later	If initial colonoscopy clear then repeat at age 55 years

Key: FAP, familial adenomatous polyposis; FDR, first-degree relative (sibling, parent or child) with colorectal cancer (CRC); HNPCC, hereditary non-polyposis colorectal cancer; IBD, inflammatory bowel disease; LFTs, liver function tests; MMR, mismatch repair gene; OGD, oesophago-gastroduodenoscopy; OLT, orthoptic liver transplantation; PSC, primary sclerosing cholangitis.

*The Amsterdam criteria for identifying HNPCC are: three or more relatives with colorectal cancer; one patient a first-degree relative of another; two generations with cancer; and one cancer diagnosed below the age of 50. The above family groups are for a minimum number of affected relatives – lifetime risk rises with additional relatives in other generations and with younger onset of disease. These guidelines assume complete colonoscopy; if incomplete then either immediate double-contrast barium enema or planned repeat colonoscopy. Note that family history may be falsely negative. People with symptoms suggestive of colorectal cancer or polyps should be appropriately investigated; they are not candidates for screening. This summary has been compiled by Cairns and Scholefield (2002). (Adapted and reproduced with permission from the BMJ Publishing Group.)

consistency is predictable. Similar guidelines have been produced by the WHO, in collaboration with the Memorial Sloan–Kettering Cancer Center (Winnawer et al. 1995). Although the nature of some family history data is not entirely reliable, currently those with a family history suggestive of a 1 in 10 lifetime risk are not usually eligible (Cairns and Scholefield 2002).

Adenocarcinoma is the phrase used to explain cancers affecting the epithelial layers of the large bowel which account for an estimated 90–95% of all cases diagnosed (DoH 1999). Adenomas are benign; any that are identified as having a 'critical' histology will require surgical treatment. Data propose that between 67 and 90% of these cases will reveal a genetic predisposition to bowel cancer. These patients are at increased risk of developing CRC, so regular surveillance after polyp removal is essential. Most adenomas would not be detected with a national CRC screening programme, although reports suggest that significant changes should be seen in this situation (Atkin and Saunders 2002).

On the whole there are two highly penetrant, autosomal dominant, predisposition syndromes: hereditary non-polyposis colorectal cancer (HNPCC) and familial adenomatous polyposis (FAP). Together they account for 2–10% of all CRCs. Confirmed HNPCC and FAP families should be registered in regional clinical genetic centres and all family members made aware of available counselling services (see Chapter 1).

Other conditions within the high-risk group include the following:

- Ulcerative colitis (UC) diagnosed at < 25 years of age with total colon involvement for 8+ years and left-sided colitis for 15 years from onset of symptoms.
- Patients with colonic Crohn's disease pose similar risks; surveillance guidelines are comparable to those for UC.
- Acromegaly – a rare condition characterized by high levels of growth hormone – is now known to increase the incidence of adenomas and CRCs (Jenkins and Fairclough 2002).
- A previous history of adenoma, colon cancer or female-specific cancers is also a recognized consideration (Cancer Research Campaign 1999) (Table 2.2).

Implications for health professionals

Increasingly more people are becoming health conscious. *The Health of the Nation* document (DoH 1992) specified targets for the promotion of good health and the prevention of ill-health. An ageing population generates additional demands on health-care provision. Health services traditionally used a medically oriented model with focus on an illness-based society and nursing care. The tide is now changing; health professionals (HPs), especially those nurses working in primary care settings, specialist and advanced practice, have increased involvement with relatively healthy people. Interventions are designed to increase levels of public health by raising awareness of active health-promotion initiatives, information, surveillance and support. Based on an individual's own health beliefs and knowledge of CRC and screening, they empower the individual to take responsibility for his or her own health. An individual's belief about the significance of and vulnerability to disease, which can trigger changes to lifestyle and behaviour, is more likely to have an effect. Factors influencing compliance include education of self and peers, and communication among HPs, patients, and voluntary and statutory agencies about bowel cancer awareness campaigns to ensure optimal programme effectiveness.

A CRC screening programme is to be welcomed in the UK. However, if the government is to establish nationwide screening, additional training requirements need to be assessed to assist with the demand and management of colorectal neoplasia. Programme implementation will require an increased clinical workforce within primary and secondary care.

Endoscopy services for existing NHS patients in the UK are already depleted in medical personnel; a screening programme will further jeopardize these services. Increasingly, nurses are seen as a key resource and, given the appropriate education and training, they are capable of working as experts in their specific areas of practice.

The advanced nurse practitioner (ANP) in endoscopy has been mentioned in reports about future workforce planning (Richards 2002). Encouraging results in a Cancer Research UK trial indicate that specially trained nurses could clearly fulfil this role; this is demonstrated by nurse endoscopists in the USA. Clinical effectiveness in endoscopic and clinical practice is established in the UK, with the evolving role of developing advanced practice. To encourage sustained programme funding and secure the effectiveness of new nursing roles, nursing research and development are vital to inform all nursing intervention.

Summary of key points

- Colorectal cancer mortality will not be reduced without heightened public awareness of early detection, screening tests, disease-associated risks and a multidisciplinary approach.
- Early detection of CRC may result in cure, and frequently a reduction in the amount or kind of treatment needed.

- Health professionals, especially those working in primary care, should assist CRC awareness programmes by developing and integrating the health belief model at every opportunity.
- Care should be focused on health promotion and disease prevention.
- Evidence suggests that action on a range of fronts is required within and outside the NHS at local, regional and national levels; this should be interpreted in the context of local need, circumstances and resources (Health Development Agency 2002).
- Collaboration between the NHS and voluntary and statutory organizations, by multiprofessional teams working in primary and secondary care, can lead to the design of services conducive to effective health improvement work.
- The implication of cancer is not only equated with mortality rates; the consequences of disease have a measurable effect on a patient's quality of life and that of his or her significant others.

References

American Cancer Society (1999) Colorectal Cancer. Atlanta, GA: ACS.
American Cancer Society (2003) Cancer facts and figures: www.cancer.org/eprise/main/docroot/STT/content/STT_1x_Cancer_Facts_Figures_2003 (accessed 20 September 2003).
Atkin WS, Saunders BP (2002) Surveillance guidelines after removal of colorectal adenomatous polyps. Gut 51(suppl V): 6-9.
Atkin WS, Cook CF, Cuzick R et al. (2002) Single flexible sigmoidoscopy screening to prevent colorectal cancer: baseline findings of a UK multicentre randomised trial. The Lancet 359: 1291-300.
Becker MH (1974) The Health Belief Model and Personal Behaviour. Thorofare, NJ: Slack.
Burkitt DP (1969) Related disease-related cause. The Lancet ii: 1229-31.
Cairns S, Scholefield JH (2002) Guidelines for colorectal cancer screening in high risk groups. Gut 51(suppl V): 1-5.
Cancer Research Campaign (1999) The Facts: Common cancers: www.cancerscreening.nhs.uk/colorectal/end-of-pilot.html.
Chamberlain J (1995) Screening for colorectal cancer. In: Chamberlain J, Moss S (eds), Evaluation of Cancer Screening. London: Springer.
Chao A, Thun MJ, Jacobs EJ et al. (2000) Cigarette smoking and cancer mortality in the cancer prevention study 11. Journal of the National Cancer Institute 92: 1888-96.
Colon Cancer Concern (2003) Viewpoint: Colon cancer road show. Cancer Nursing Practice 2: 16-17
Cummings JH, Bingham SA (1998) Diet and the prevention of cancer. British Medical Journal 317: 1636-40
Department of Health (1992) The Health of the Nation: A strategy for health in England. London: The Stationery Office.
Department of Health (1997-98) Committee on Medical Aspects of Food Policy (COMA). London: The Stationery Office.
Department of Health (1999) Saving Lives: Our healthier nation. London: The Stationery Office.

De Snoo L (2003) Colorectal cancer. Primary Health Care 13(3): 43–9.

Dominitz JA, Provenzale D (1997) Patient preferences and quality of life associated with colorectal cancer screening. American Journal of Gastroenterology 92: 2171–8.

Downie RS, Fyfe C, Tannahill A (1996) Health Promotion Models and Values, 2nd edn. Oxford: Oxford University Press.

Gott M, O'Brien M (1990) The role of the nurse in health promotion: policies, perspectives and practice. European Journal of Cancer Care 28: 1–3.

Hardcastle J, Chamberlain J, Robinson M et al. (1996) Randomised controlled trial of faecal occult blood test. The Lancet 348: 1472–7.

Hart AR, Wicks ACB, Mayberry JF (1995) Colorectal cancer screening in asymptomatic populations. Gut 36: 590–8.

Health Development Agency (2002) Cancer Prevention: A resource to support local action in delivering the NHS Cancer Plan. London: HDA.

Health Promotion Authority for Wales (1990) Health for All in Wales: Strategies for action. Cardiff: Health Promotion Authority for Wales

Heller T, Davey B, Bailey C (1989) Reducing the Risk of Cancers. London: Hodder & Stoughton.

Janne PA, Mayer RJ (2001) Chemoprevention of colorectal cancer. New England Journal of Medicine 342: 1960–8.

Jenkins PJ, Fairclough PD (2002) Screening guidelines for colorectal cancer and polyps in patients with acromegaly. Gut 51(suppl V): 13–14.

Kim Y (2000) AGA technical review: impact of dietary fiber on colon cancer occurrence. Gastroenterology 118: 1235–57.

Kronberg O, Fenger C, Olsen J et al. (1996) Randomised controlled study of screening for colorectal cancer with faecal occult blood test. The Lancet 348: 1467–71.

Lindholm E, Bergland B, Kerwinter J et al. (1997) Worry associated with screening for colorectal carcinomas. Scandinavian Journal of Gastroenterology 32: 230–45.

Mandel JS, Church TR, Ederer F et al. (1999) Colorectal cancer mortality: effectiveness of biennial screening for fecal occult blood. Journal of National Cancer Institute 91: 434–7.

Midgley R, Kerr D (1999) Colorectal cancer. The Lancet 353: 391–9.

National Cancer Guidance Steering Group (2004) Improving Outcomes in Colorectal Cancer: Manual update. London: NICE.

NHS (2003) NHS Bowel Cancer programme: Launch of a new programme of work to tackle bowel cancer. Press release, 4 February. London: Department of Health: www:info.doh.gov.uk/doh/intpress.nsf (last accessed 12 January 2004).

NHS Centre for Reviews and Dissemination (1997) Effective Health Care: The management of colorectal cancer. York: University of York.

NHS Executive (1997) Guidance on Commissioning Cancer Services: Improving outcomes in colorectal cancer: The research evidence. London: Department of Health.

Northern Ireland Department of Health and Social Security (1991) A Regional Strategy for the Northern Ireland Health and Personal Social Services 1992–1997. Belfast: NIDHSS

Pender NJ, Murdaugh CL, Parsons MA (2002) Empowering for self-care across a lifespan. In: Conner M (ed.), Health Promotion in Nursing Practice, 4th edn. Upper Saddle River, NJ: Prentice Hall.

Rawl SB, Menon U, Champion V (2002) Colorectal screening: an overview of current trends. Nursing Clinics of North America 37: 225–45.

Richards M (2002) News: Nurses could play a key role in screening for colorectal cancer. Nursing Times 98(46): 6.

Scottish Office (1992) Scotland's Health: A challenge to us all. Edinburgh: HMSO.

Scottish Office Home and Health Department (1991) Health Education in Scotland: A national policy statement. Edinburgh: The Scottish Office.

Tannahill A (1985) What is health promotion? Health Education Journal 44: 167–8

Terry P, Giovannucci EL, Michel KB et al. (2001) Fruit, vegetables, dietary fiber, and risk of colorectal cancer. Journal of the National Cancer Institute 93: 525–33.

Towler B, Irwig L, Glasziou P et al. (1998) A systematic review of the effects of screening for colorectal cancer using faecal occult blood test, Haemoccult. British Medical Journal 317: 559–65.

Tuswell AS (2002) Meat consumption and cancer of the large bowel. European Journal of Clinical Nutrition 56(suppl 1): 519–24.

Viewpoint (2003) Colon cancer road show. Cancer Nursing Practice 2(2): 16–17.

Whittaker J (2001) Colorectal cancer. In: Gabriel J (ed.), Oncology Nursing Practice. London: Whurr Publishers.

Winnawer SJ, St John DJ, Bond JH et al. (1995) Prevention of Colorectal Cancer: Guidelines based on new data. Geneva: WHO.

World Health Organization (1946) Constitution. New York: WHO.

World Health Organization (1978) Alma-Ata Report on Primary Health Care. Geneva: WHO.

World Health Organization (1984) Health Promotion: A discussion document on the concept and principles. Copenhagen: WHO.

Further reading

Downie RS, Fyfe C, Tannahill A (1996) Health Promotion Models and Values, 2nd edn. Oxford: Oxford University Press

Useful websites

www.crc.org.uk/cancer/aboutcan_common.3html
www.info@cancerscreening.nhs.uk
www.statistics.gov.uk

Chapter 3

Diagnosis and staging

Barry Rawlings and Barbara Borwell

The recognition of the early clinical features of any cancer is seen as important. Such recognition may lead not only to a reduction of mortality, but also to prevention of some of the more distressing aspects of morbidity associated with the more advanced, albeit treatable, cancers. Colorectal carcinoma is unlikely to be an exception, although some workers question whether early diagnosis of symptoms of this particular cancer leads to improved survival (Thompson et al. 2003). Such debate, however, must be set alongside national guidance on the importance of referral and investigation in colorectal cancer (NHS Executive 1997a, 1997b, National Cancer Guidance Steering Group or NCGSG 2004). In any event, we should not be deflected from acknowledging our need for awareness of early clinical presentations of colorectal cancer.

Naturally, no firm diagnosis can be made without the aid of a physical examination, in which a digital rectal examination is mandatory, and a battery of investigations, some of which can be carried out at the bedside while others require the services of the endoscopy, imaging and pathology departments of a hospital. Although many readers have no responsibility for conducting physical examinations or ordering investigations, such matters may be of interest to them.

In addition, staging procedures will be needed in order to ascertain the extent to which the carcinoma has invaded the bowel wall and spread to other sites. Staging, which is based on clinical, imaging and intraoperative information, should not be confused with grading; the latter is the responsibility of the histopathologist who, by microscopic examination, characterizes the tumour's level of aggressiveness from observation of its cellular components and activity. It is not appropriate for this chapter to give any further coverage of grading.

Clinical features

In considering the clinical features of bowel cancer, it is useful to start by reminding ourselves of the 'adenoma–carcinoma sequence' (see Chapter 1). Adenomatous polyps, which have malignant potential, may give rise to symptoms, as may those that constitute the rare familial polyposis syndromes. An example of the latter group is familial adenomatous polyposis (FAP), a condition that is often known about before any symptoms arise because it is usual for members of afflicted families to undergo regular screening from adolescence onwards. Unusual though it may be for the 'adenoma phase' of the sequence to cause symptoms, we should note the clinical features that could arise in that phase. It needs to be said at this point that, because of the relative rarity of symptoms in the phase, it is difficult to ascribe to any one feature its relative frequency of appearance in a patient. The health professional who follows good practice will, however, ensure that the cause of any of the features described in this chapter is established and not simply assumed, without appropriate investigation, to be caused by haemorrhoids, stress, dietary change or indiscretion, even though these common situations can be associated with some of those features. Some of the possible clinical features of the 'adenoma phase' are:

- rectal bleeding
- anaemia
- mucus discharge, at, or separate from, the act of defecation
- loose stools
- tenesmus (referring to a frequent desire to defecate with little, if any, result, despite painful straining).

Moving to a detailed consideration of the possible clinical features that may appear in patients in whom the 'carcinoma phase' of the sequence has been reached, the features described can also be expected in situations where colorectal carcinoma has developed in the absence of any obvious 'adenoma–carcinoma sequence'. It is worth reiterating the view concerning good practice. Signs and symptoms of the kind we often see in early colorectal carcinoma can too easily be dismissed as being caused by common and non-threatening situations such as haemorrhoids, etc. 'Common things occur commonly' is a useful aphorism and it is a fact that haemorrhoids do occur commonly and are high on the list of likely causes for blood on the faeces. However, we ignore, at the patient's peril, relatively less likely causes, such as carcinoma of the rectosigmoid region.

We should not overlook other aspects of the patient's history. A previous bowel cancer increases the risk of a second tumour, for example, and ulcerative colitis responding poorly to drug therapy over a long period of time increases the risk of colorectal cancer. A family history of bowel cancer is also a recognized risk factor.

Many both within and beyond the health-care professions consider carcinoma (of any organ) to be a disease of the older person. Although this belief is valid in general terms, it undoubtedly will not be difficult for the reader to call to mind cases of relatively young patients with a solid tumour malignancy such as colorectal cancer. This particular cancer is occasionally seen in quite young adults, although the more usual presenting age is from about 50 years onwards (Mortensen 2000, Williams 2000). There is no universal agreement on a minimum age at which it is mandatory to investigate patients complaining of clinical features that could be associated with colorectal cancer. One could argue a case for investigating all such patients, although the economics of this approach would be problematic. Some might be happy to agree with those who suggest investigation should be initiated in patients aged 35–40 years and beyond (Clark and Silk 2002). Whatever the view taken, it is certain that such debate will be sterile unless we are fully aware of the possible clinical presentations, i.e. the signs and symptoms exhibited and experienced by patients, of this type of cancer. Without an awareness of the possible significance of these signs and symptoms there is little likelihood of a professional moving on to think of initiating investigations. So we must look at what the patient may tell us and what we may see on our assessment.

In considering the early clinical features of colorectal cancer, it is essential to realize that how the tumour presents will depend on its location within the large intestine. It is of some (but not much) comfort, perhaps, to note that the more insidious features are most often associated with the tumours that make up only about 25% of all colorectal cancers (see Chapter 1). It is, however, those very features that can, because of their 'vague' nature, easily be overlooked or dismissed by either patient or professional.

The more noticeable features, by their very nature being more likely to be picked up and explored, are usually associated with the more common sites of colorectal carcinoma. It has to be accepted, however, that some patients with even the most florid symptoms will delay weeks or months before presenting themselves for professional consultation. In this situation, as in so many in the field of health, the whole matter of outcome, in terms of both morbidity and mortality, depends on the patient's behaviour. Health education is surely vital in encouraging the appropriate behaviour on the part of patients.

Crawford (1999) suggests that 25–30% of patients with colorectal carcinoma are found at the time of diagnosis to be beyond the help of curative surgery. This situation is no doubt partly the result of patients' late presentations, but also an outcome of missed or delayed diagnosis.

The matter of health education, which could help the former, cannot be addressed here, but the latter can. The following account is offered in the hope of raising our index of suspicion when considering the possibility of underlying carcinoma in any of the regions of the large bowel.

It is convenient to divide the large bowel into three areas (Figure 3.1):

- Right-sided
- Left-sided
- Rectosigmoid.

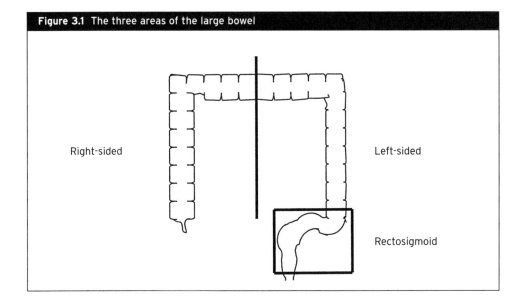

Figure 3.1 The three areas of the large bowel

Right-sided

- Anaemia
- Weight loss: a late feature
- Palpable mass: also a late feature.

A carcinoma may cause a patient to present with complaints of continual tiredness, fatigue or weakness. Such symptoms will result from anaemia which, in turn, is caused by the fact that right-sided carcinomas are bulky tumours that can bleed easily (Crawford 1999). Such bleeding is invariably minimal and so the type of anaemia will be that of iron deficiency. It is a common mistake to view iron deficiency anaemia as being caused simply by a lack of dietary iron. This is an unusual cause in the UK. It is safer to assume that, until proved otherwise, all such anaemias are the result of some underlying chronic, albeit relatively small, blood loss. Other causes of this type of anaemia can of course be related to malabsorption in the small bowel caused, for example, by Crohn's disease. Another common misconception about anaemia (of any type) is that it always manifests itself with all the signs and symptoms reported in textbooks, such as facial pallor, spoon-shaped nails (koilonychia), pale palmar creases, dyspnoea, etc. (Talley and O'Connor 1996). Usually only patients with severe anaemia display a full list of signs and symptoms! Complaints of tiredness, coupled with pale conjunctivae, should be enough to set us thinking of anaemia. We then need to establish the cause of the anaemia, remembering that anaemia is not a diagnosis in itself.

Weight loss is well known as a feature of most carcinomatous situations and colorectal cancer is no exception. Lipid and muscle cells are lost, i.e. both fat and lean body mass are reduced. Such weight loss is thought to be the result of the action of certain protein substances, known as 'cytokines', being secreted by inflammatory cells present in parts of the cancer (Stevens and Lowe 2000).

During physical examination by a doctor or nurse practitioner the tumour, if sufficiently large, may be felt by deep palpation of the right side of the abdomen.

Left-sided

- Alteration in bowel habit
- Blood mixed in with faeces
- Colicky abdominal pain: a later feature
- Lower abdominal distension: also, usually, a later feature
- Weight loss: a later feature
- Palpable mass: also, a later feature.

It matters less in which way bowel habit alters than the fact that there has been an alteration. It is often, but by no means always, the case that there are increasing problems of constipation, such episodes being followed by bouts of diarrhoea. Nevertheless, any adult with previously regular defecation routines who develops irregularity of habit – regardless of whether this involves constipation or loose stools – should always be regarded as a possible candidate for a left-sided bowel carcinoma. It is essential, however, for both patient and practitioner to have a joint understanding of what precisely each of them means by terms such as 'constipation' and 'diarrhoea' because there are wildly varying interpretations.

To what extent blood mixes in with faeces is largely governed by the location of the left-sided tumour. A cancer in the left transverse colon or proximal descending colon is likely to present with well-mixed blood.

Dark-coloured stools may be passed but, as bleeding is usually minimal, there may be no colour change and investigation for occult blood will be necessary. A tumour in the distal descending colon or sigmoid flexure is more likely to show itself as fresher-looking blood with little mixing into the faeces.

Many left-sided carcinomas are of the stenosing type (Mortensen 2000); such narrowing arises from the fact that the tumour encircles the gut wall and can form what has been referred to as a 'napkin-ring' constriction (Crawford 1999). This type of lesion can give rise to symptoms of progressive bowel obstruction, of which colicky pain is likely to be the main one. Pain of this nature is caused by stretching and contraction of a hollow organ, i.e. a viscus (Grace and Borley 2002). Hence, such a pain is often called 'visceral' pain. The viscus here is the left colon which undergoes vigorous peristalsis in its efforts to clear gut contents through the stenosed region. Success in this effort of clearance is usually signalled by relief from pain. The pain is often poorly localized and, being visceral, tends to be referred to the middle of the abdomen and, as distal colon is involved, over the suprapubic region (Welsby 1996). It must be pointed out that the feature of pain is probably to be expected at a slightly later stage of the carcinoma's development. It must also be noted that, should pain be constant, rather than colicky, it is likely that the tumour is at a fairly advanced stage.

Distension in the lower abdominal region may be seen by the examining practitioner. It is caused by gas accumulation above the stenosed area and so is relieved by the passing of flatus. Again it needs to be appreciated that this particular feature forms part of the picture of partial gut obstruction and so is more likely to occur at a rather later stage of the disease.

Weight loss and palpation of an abdominal mass are both late features and the comments made above when discussing right-sided carcinomas apply equally to left-sided ones. The obvious exception, of course, is that any palpable mass will be situated somewhere in the left abdomen.

Rectosigmoid

- Rectal bleeding
- Alteration in bowel habit
- Mucus discharge at defecation
- Tenesmus
- Palpable mass: a late feature *or* an early feature (see discussion below)
- Pain: variable in site and nature, but usually a late feature
- Weight loss: a late feature.

Bleeding is usually the earliest feature. It may be only slight but must be explored appropriately. The blood is fresh, i.e. bright red in colour, and may be seen with the faeces or at the end of a defecation episode. Some patients will comment on the presence of blood stains on their under-clothes and this can suggest either poor cleansing routines post-defecation or that the bleeding is severe enough to occur also between defecation episodes. When one learns that 97% of patients in primary care with rec-tal bleeding do not have colorectal carcinoma (Thompson et al. 2003), it is, as mentioned earlier, very easy to assume haemorrhoids to be the cause of the bleeding. It cannot be reiterated too many times that such an assumption is totally unwarranted without further exploration of the sit-uation. It also needs to be constantly borne in mind by health-care professionals that haemorrhoids, even when found on examination or proctoscopy, can coexist with rectosigmoid carcinoma. The carcinoma can compress, and even cause thrombosis in, some veins in that area, which can give rise to the varicosities we call haemorrhoids (Williams 2000). It is therefore necessary to use the proctoscope to its fullest extent by examining as much of the rectum as possible; indeed, many would argue for the use of a rigid sigmoidoscope, if not a flexible one, because high rectal carcinomas can be missed if only proctoscopy is undertaken.

Altered bowel habit is also an early feature of rectosigmoid cancer. As with other large bowel tumours, whether constipation or looseness is the presenting problem is immaterial. The fact that a change in habit has occurred is the point on which one must focus. For interest, however, it can be said that a tumour in the proximal rectum is more likely to give rise to constipation and one in the mid- to lower rectum tends more to cause diar-rhoeal features (Williams 2000), the latter often being particularly troublesome in the early morning. Care must be taken when questioning patients in order to avoid confusion over the type of alteration in bowel habit that they have been experiencing; it is possible that they suffered con-stipation symptoms and consequently treated them themselves with 'over-the-counter' laxatives, which may have resulted in loose stools being passed and described by the patient in terms of diarrhoea.

Mucus, sometimes described as slime, is often an accompaniment to the faeces and blood passed by patients. Again, it has to be realized that mucus discharge is a not unusual feature in haemorrhoids, especially those with a tendency to prolapse.

Tenesmus, defined earlier, is an unpleasant and often uncomfortable symptom which can give patients a sense of incomplete defecation where-by they open their bowels to a greater or lesser extent but feel that there are more faeces to be expelled; no expulsion of faecal material occurs, however, because there is no such material left in the rectum. It is a par-ticularly common feature of tumours located in the lower rectum.

Palpation should be performed on the lower abdomen in every patient complaining of the features discussed here. It is only if the tumour is in the sigmoid or high rectal region, and is at an advanced stage of development, that there will be any chance of palpating the mass. It can therefore be concluded that a positive finding of this kind on abdominal palpation indicates a poor prognosis for the patient. By way of contrast, digital rectal examination can be a means of detecting an early rectal carcinoma, particularly one situated in the mid- or lower rectum. It is beyond the scope of this chapter to discuss the techniques of palpation, of either the abdomen or the rectum. Suffice it to remind ourselves that no digital examination of the rectum would be complete without inspecting the gloved finger on withdrawal for blood or mucus mixed with blood. Such blood may well have derived from contact by the finger with a bleeding haemorrhoid but, equally, that contact may have been with a cancer.

Constant pain is not a feature of rectal carcinoma, as a rule, until a late stage has been reached. Colicky pain, however, may occur in cases of partial obstruction of the sigmoid colon or of the junction of the latter with the rectum.

Carcinoma of the anal canal and anus

It is perhaps worth making brief mention of carcinoma in this region. Carcinoma of the anal canal is rare but can give rise to clinical features that are similar to those found in cancer of the rectosigmoid area. An additional symptom may be the feeling of having a solid object in the anal canal. Carcinoma of the anus, i.e. the opening of the anal canal to the external body, is even rarer than that of the canal and shows itself as a form of skin cancer.

A detailed account of the clinical features of colorectal cancer has been offered for the simple reason that most readers are likely to be in a position to listen to, and ask questions of, patients giving their histories. It is therefore vital to possess a sound understanding that can reveal the significance of what we hear and see when assessing patients.

Although it is important that readers understand investigations that may follow provisional or firm diagnosis, it is unlikely that many will be initiating such investigations or interpreting their results. It is intended therefore to address these topics in rather less detail than was given for clinical features. Only investigations related directly to the gut are covered; blood tests to show, for example, anaemia from bleeding or liver problems from metastases are not addressed below.

Investigations

Faecal occult blood testing

Faecal occult blood testing (FOBT) is required when right-sided colon cancer is suspected or unexplained anaemia is found. The sensitivity of FOBT is a matter of debate and can vary with the laboratory method used. Most studies suggest that only 60% or less of patients with colonic carcinoma will show a positive result on FOBT, so there will be a significant number of 'false-negative' results. Patients in the 'adenoma phase' are even less likely to be detected by FOBT. The test is more successful in excluding bowel cancer, however, because it gives a (correct) negative result in about 90% or more of individuals who do not have the disease (Nattinger 1999). This means that there are few 'false-positive' results in FOBT and so it has a high specificity, in contrast to its sensitivity.

To summarize, a positive FOBT is very likely to be obtained in a patient with colon cancer. A negative result cannot be used definitively to exclude such a diagnosis. Two further points, however, must be borne in mind. First, other gastrointestinal disorders may involve bleeding and therefore give a positive FOBT result. Second, the patient must be adequately prepared in terms of dietary restriction before submitting faecal specimens for FOBT. With all these points in mind, a case can easily be made for omitting FOBT and proceeding directly to other investigations which offer higher sensitivity (and equal, or even better, specificity).

Radiology

Double-contrast barium enema, in which air and barium are administered, has a high sensitivity and specificity for carcinoma, and also for adenomatous polyps of a centimetre or more (Nattinger 1999). Use as a diagnostic tool will decline as endoscopy services expand (NCGSG 2004). Rigorous bowel preparation is required for this investigation.

Endoscopy

Mention has already been made of proctoscopy and sigmoidoscopy. No bowel preparation is required for the former, or for the latter when using a rigid sigmoidoscope (beyond the obvious need for the rectum to be empty). The proctoscope can reach to about 10 cm from the anus and so offer a view of the lower rectum. The rigid sigmoidoscope can reach to about 20 cm or so and therefore can allow one to visualize the whole rectum but only the distal sigmoid colon. Both instruments are often made of Perspex and so are disposable. The flexible sigmoidoscope is not, however, disposable although, reaching to 60 cm as it does, it can offer views of the entire sigmoid colon. Bowel preparation is required so that the region is devoid of faeces.

Such preparation (though of a rather more rigorous nature) is also required for colonoscopy. Sedation is also used in this procedure. This form of endoscopy, which visualizes the large bowel in its entirety, is often regarded as the 'gold standard' test for detecting colon cancer. Its sensitivity and specificity are very high (90–100%) for both cancer and polyps (Nattinger 1999).

Although we are focusing on the use of these investigations in a situation where a patient has already complained of symptoms, it is worth noting here that the charity Cancer Research UK is calling for national screening for bowel cancer by means of mass flexible sigmoidoscopy and FOBT. The charity estimates that about 5000 lives a year could be saved in this way (Iles 2003). The reader must judge the limitations of the two investigations suggested and the costs of the programme against the predicted gains in lives saved.

Other investigations

After diagnosis by one or more of the above means, ultrasonography, computed tomography (CT) or magnetic resonance imaging (MRI) may be used to assess the size of the tumour as well as to detect both local and metastatic spread. Advances in radiology technology clearly extend the capabilities of other imaging modalities. Positron emission tomography (PET) produces images of molecular level physiological function where physicians can identify abnormal states, offering unique diagnostic information. Already used in some major institutions, this, in the future, may alter patient management in oncology (National PET Scan Management 2004).

In some cancers, colorectal carcinoma included, certain chemicals are released from the tumour cells into the blood. Some of these tumour markers, as they are called, are normally released only from foetal, but not adult, cells whereas other markers are released in greater amounts from tumour cells than from normal cells. Although these markers may aid diagnosis, their main use at present is in monitoring the response to treatment of the cancer. A substance known as carcinoma embryonic antigen (CEA) can be found in the blood of patients with colorectal carcinoma in 60–90% of cases. It should be noted that CEA levels can rise in other cancers and in some non-malignant diseases, and so this test is probably better used for monitoring treatment response, although it appears that pre-treatment levels of CEA can indicate the extent of the cancer; and CEA levels do correlate well with the Dukes' staging system (Cotran et al. 1999).

Staging of a tumour gives an indication of the extent of growth and spread and the Dukes' system of staging has been in use for many years. In 1932 Cuthbert Dukes, a London pathologist, produced his staging scheme for rectal cancers only, but the system has been applied to carcinomas in the large bowel generally. This broader usage has involved various modifications being made and so it is always necessary to check which particular version has been used for a patient (Stevens and Lowe 2000). The Dukes' scheme is considered to be simple, reproducible and accurate in indicating prognosis (surgical-tutor.org.uk 2003). An example of the scheme is given in Figure 3.2. Dukes' original scheme did not include a 'D' category, but others have added it to signify metastases in distant organs.

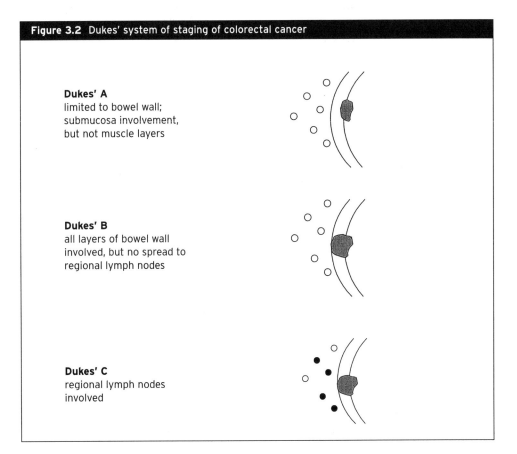

Figure 3.2 Dukes' system of staging of colorectal cancer

Dukes' A
limited to bowel wall; submucosa involvement, but not muscle layers

Dukes' B
all layers of bowel wall involved, but no spread to regional lymph nodes

Dukes' C
regional lymph nodes involved

The Dukes' system may become less favoured (Clark and Silk 2002) because the International Union Against Cancer's TNM scheme for staging offers a more detailed classification of cancers, colorectal cancer being no exception. The three letters represent tumour, nodes and metastases, so the system assesses the extent of the tumour's local spread (invasion), the regional lymph node involvement and the presence of metastases in distant organs. The resulting information is scored. An outline of the scheme is depicted in Figure 3.3.

Figure 3.3 TNM staging

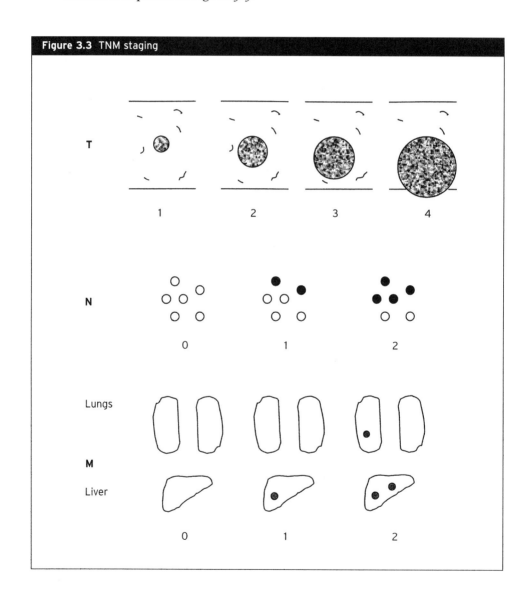

The T number is governed by the tumour size and the extent of its invasion of the various layers of the bowel wall. The N number is decided by the number and range of lymph nodes enlarged, and their tissue replaced, by tumour cells. The pattern of lymph node involvement is related to the normal routes of drainage of lymph from the organ containing the tumour. The M number refers to the extent of metastasis, i.e. secondary spread to distant organs. The last can occur not only through the lymphatic system but also via the bloodstream, the portal vein being the route of spread when we come across the common finding of liver metastases in advanced colorectal carcinoma.

Once a diagnosis has been confirmed by the investigations discussed earlier and the staging and grading procedures have been carried out, conclusions can be drawn concerning the likely prognosis, and decisions can be made about appropriate treatment.

In view of the stage-related prognosis, early diagnosis of colorectal cancer is essential. Evidence suggests that, at the time of presentation of symptoms, the cancer may be at an advanced stage (NHS Executive 1997a, see also Chapter 2). The quality of diagnostic services, including adequate endoscopy facilities, is imperative, not only for symptomatic diagnosis but also for surveillance in those patients who are at increased risk of developing colorectal cancer. Rapid access to endoscopy services should be available for all general practitioners for the prompt evaluation of suggestive signs and symptoms. Cancer networks need to monitor waiting time to endoscopy if they are to achieve the proposed 2-month standard from urgent GP referral to treatment by 2005 (NCGSG 2004). Hobbs (2000) reported detrimental differences in survival rates between England and Wales and the rest of western Europe for colorectal cancer arise within the first 6 months of diagnosis, and that these differences are related to either late presentation or delays in treatment.

The Calman–Hine Report (Expert Advisory Group on Cancer 1995), a publication on the provision of cancer services, proposes that cancer care should be provided within a collaborative network of cancer centres or units across the UK to ensure equity of access to specialized services, care and treatment. Colorectal cancer (CRC) management should be the responsibility of a CRC multidisciplinary team (MDT) consisting of core members with recognized specialist expertise, including specialist nurses with site-specific expertise (NHS Executive 1996, NCGSG 2004) to provide specialized nursing care and psychological support to a recognized standard. General guidelines produced by the United Kingdom Central Council (UKCC 1992) for the development of innovative ways of working, and the NHS Management Executive (1990) document on the reduction of junior doctors' hours, provide opportunities for role development and extension within the parameters of clinical practice. The emphasis is on the provision of high-quality care, which is responsive to individual patient/client needs (UKCC 1992). Although specialist nursing is not a recent development (Royal College of Nursing or RCN 1988, Spross and Baggerley 1989, McSharry 1995, Beecroft and Pappenhausen 1998, Castledine 1998, Armstrong 1999), the role of the specialist colorectal nurse is a relatively new concept, informed by the expansion of the stoma care nurse and advances in nursing science and technology. Their role and responsibilities may vary throughout the UK. Some colorectal nurse specialists work only with those patients diagnosed with cancer; others deal with people presenting with a range of colorectal conditions, benign or malignant, in many instances undertaking a technical role including that of screening and follow-up endoscopy.

The development of nurse-led diagnostic and rapid access clinics for bowel cancer are perceived and supported by the government because of their impact on patient waiting times after GP referral (Bundy 2002).

Other functions include health education activities, communication, the provision of information and psychological support before investigations, and after diagnosis acting as a coordinator of patient care and a central member of the MDT (NHS Executive 1997c). In fact nurses are at the forefront of initiatives to improve the UK's bowel cancer survival rates (Fursland 2004, NCGSG 2004).

Summary of key points

- It is important that health professionals are knowledgeable about the early clinical presentations of colorectal carcinoma.
- Such an awareness, when exercised in clinical practice, may enable the health-care professional to initiate a patient's entry into an appropriate assessment situation.
- Having some general understanding of the diagnostic and staging procedures used to establish the presence and extent of colorectal carcinoma is useful for health-care professionals.

References

Armstrong P (1999) The role of the clinical nurse specialist. Nursing Standard 13(16): 40-2.
Beecroft PC, Pappenhausen JL (1998) What is a specialist? Clinical Nurse Specialist 2(3): 109-12
Bundy K (2002) Comfort zone. Nursing Standard 16(19): 17-18.

Castledine G (1998) Developments in the role of the advanced nursing practitioner: a personal perspective. In: Rolfe G, Fulbrook P (eds), Advanced Nursing Practice. Oxford: Butterworth-Heinemann.

Clark ML, Silk DB (2002) Gastrointestinal disease. In: Kumar P, Clark ML (eds), Clinical Medicine, 5th edn. Edinburgh: WB Saunders, pp. 253–333.

Cotran RS, Kumar V, Collins T (1999) Robbins' Pathologic Basis of Disease, 6th edn. Philadelphia: WB Saunders.

Crawford JM (1999) The gastrointestinal tract. In: Cotran RS, Kumar V, Collins T (eds), Robbins' Pathologic Basis of Disease, 6th edn. Philadelphia: WB Saunders, pp. 775–844.

Expert Advisory Group on Cancer (1995) The Calman-Hine Report: A policy framework for commissioning cancer services. London: HMSO.

Fursland E (2004) No nonsense approach. Nursing Standard 18(29): 16–17.

Grace PA, Borley NR (2002) Surgery at a Glance, 2nd edn. Oxford: Blackwell Science.

Hobbs FA (2000) ABC of colorectal cancer: the role of primary care. British Medical Journal 321: 1068–70.

Iles A (2003) Charity recommends introduction of screening programme for bowel cancer (News extra). British Medical Journal 327: 642.

McSharry M (1995) The evolving role of the clinical nurse specialist. British Journal of Clinical Nursing 4 (11): 641–6.

Mortensen NJMcC (2000) The small and large intestines. In: Russell RCG, Williams NS, Bulstrode CJK (eds), Bailey and Love's Short Practice of Surgery, 23rd edn. London: Arnold, pp. 1026–57.

National Cancer Guidance Steering Group (2004) Improving Outcomes in Colorectal Cancer: Manual update. London: NICE.

National PET Scan Management (2004) LLC: www.nationalpetscan.com/petovew.htm (accessed 20 February 2004).

Nattinger AB (1999) Colon cancer. In: Black ER, Bordley DR, Tape TG, Panzer RJ (eds), Diagnostic Strategies for Common Medical Problems, 2nd edn. Philadelphia: American College of Physicians, pp. 140–8.

NHS Executive (1996) Improving Outcomes in Breast Cancer: The research evidence. London: NHSE.

NHS Executive (1997a) Improving Outcomes in Colorectal Cancer: The research evidence. London: Department of Health.

NHS Executive (1997b) Improving Outcomes in Colorectal Cancer: The manual. London: Department of Health.

NHS Executive (1997c) Improving Outcomes in Colorectal Cancer: Guidance on commissioning cancer services. Leeds: NHSE.

NHS Management Executive (1990) Junior Doctors: The new deal. London: NHS Management Executive.

Royal College of Nursing (1988) Specialities in Nursing: A report of the working party investigating the development of specialities within the nursing profession. London: RCN.

Spross JA, Baggerley J (1989) Models of advanced nursing practice. In: Hamric AB, Spross JA (eds), The Clinical Nurse Specialist in Theory and Practice, 2nd edn. Philadelphia, PA: WB Saunders, pp. 19–40.

Stevens A, Lowe J (2000) Pathology, 2nd edn. Edinburgh: Mosby.

surgical-tutor.org.uk (2003).

Talley NJ, O'Connor S (1996) Clinical Examination, 3rd edn. Oxford: Blackwell Science.

Thompson MR et al. (2003) Identifying and managing patients at low risk of bowel cancer in general practice. British Medical Journal 327: 263–5.

United Kingdom Central Council (1992) The Scope of Professional Practice. London: UKCC.

Welsby PD (1996) Clinical History Taking and Examination. Edinburgh: Churchill Livingstone.

Williams NS (2000) The rectum. In: Russell RCG, Williams NS, Bulstrode CJK (eds), Bailey and Love's Short Practice of Surgery, 23rd edn. London: Arnold, pp. 1093–114.

Further reading

Phillips J, Murray P, Kirk P (eds) (2001) The Biology of Disease, 2nd edn. Oxford: Blackwell Science, Chapter 24.

Russell RCG, Williams NS, Bulstrode CJK (eds) (2000) Bailey and Love's Short Practice of Surgery, 23rd edn. London: Arnold, Chapters 57, 58 and 60.

Thompson MR et al. (2003) Identifying and managing patients at low risk of bowel cancer in general practice. British Medical Journal 327: 263-5.

Also of interest

'Rapid Responses' to above (bmj.com – issue for 2 August 2003 www.doh.gov.uk/cancer/colorectal.htm).

Part 2

The treatment of bowel cancer

Chapter 4

Background to practice

Tanya Andrewes

This chapter outlines the key drivers for change in cancer care services and explores the implications for health-care professionals in relation to service improvement strategies and education requirements.

The condition of cancer poses a significant health problem in the UK, overtaking coronary heart disease as the leading cause of mortality in the late 1990s (Tattersall and Thomas 1999), and accounting for significant use of health service resources (Dunlop 1997). Since the 1990s cancer care has been an area receiving a focus for attention in relation to developing more effective services for patients (Expert Advisory Group on Cancer 1995), alongside other key health areas such as mental health (Department of Health or DoH 1999), diabetes (DoH 2001a) and care of the older person (DoH 2001b). Although cancer remains a serious, potentially life-threatening problem, the significant advances in therapeutic treatment over the last decade have resulted in more effective management, with cure in some cases. Side effects are no longer deemed to be inevitable and those that present are effectively managed, in most cases, by a range of therapeutic interventions.

A major government audit into cancer morbidity and mortality rates in the UK in the early 1990s revealed that one in three people develop cancer and one in four die as a result of the disease (Expert Advisory Group on Cancer 1995). A further outcome of the audit was the revelation of a picture of statistically significant differences in mortality rates when comparing treatment centres across the UK, and when comparing the UK with the rest of the world. The subsequent report (Expert Advisory Group on Cancer 1995) represented the first National Service Framework and set out a number of recommendations for improvement and change that would serve to enhance cancer services, throughout every aspect of the cancer journey from health promotion and illness prevention, through screening, diagnosis and treatment, to resolution or a peaceful and supported death. This included the proposal for the delivery of cancer care services through a network of cancer centres and cancer units, working together to ensure equity of access to patients and their carers, as close to the home as possible, and with equity measured in terms of treatment outcomes. The report also served as a substantial driver for the widespread development and provision of accredited specialist education to healthcare professionals as a means of improving cancer care services.

Strategies for developing good practice

Colorectal cancer is one type of cancer that has received specific attention in terms of the improvement of cancer care services (NHS Executive 2000). Notably, colorectal cancer incidence accounts for the fourth most common cancer on a worldwide scale (Boyle 1998), and was recorded as the second most common cancer in both the male and the female population in the UK in 1999 (Cancer Research UK 2003a). In terms of mortality, even though the overall number of deaths has fallen over the last decade, colorectal cancer still accounted for 10% of all deaths from cancer in 2001, or 16 165 deaths (Cancer Research UK 2003b), exceeded only by deaths from lung cancer. The overall survival rate from colorectal cancer is 40–45%; however, this can be increased to as much as 70% with curative surgery (Dunlop 1997). In addition, a number of screening tests have been developed to facilitate earlier diagnosis of colorectal cancer, when the disease is eminently treatable. Therefore, colorectal cancer is a justifiable focus for the improvement of services.

Subsequent to the publication of the Policy Framework for Commissioning Cancer Services (Expert Advisory Group on Cancer 1995), a number of new policy and guidance documents (DoH 2000a, NHS Executive 2000) have been published, under the guidance of a National Cancer Director to guide the further development of cancer services, including cancer networks and cancer services collaboratives (DoH 2000a, 2003a). The main influence and function of these structures, reflecting the original Policy Framework for Commissioning Cancer Services (Expert Advisory Group on Cancer 1995), and informed by the national survey of cancer patients (DoH 2002), is to continue to streamline cancer services and to develop local, regional and national policies based on the best available evidence, thus maximizing the outcomes of cancer care and treatment through a skilled and committed workforce. *The NHS Cancer Plan* (DoH 2000a), in particular, set out a comprehensive national strategy for cancer and has served as a key driver for substantial cancer services funding (DoH 2001c), in order to:

- save more lives
- ensure that people with cancer get the right professional support and care as well as the best treatments

- tackle the inequalities in health that result in a twofold mortality rate from cancer in unskilled workers when compared with professionals
- build for the future through investment in the cancer workforce, through strong research and preparation for the genetics revolution.

This plan (DoH 2000a) and the associated funding seek to ensure that NHS cancer services never fall behind again.

Improvements in colorectal cancer services are fundamentally founded on the application of evidence-based practices through the development and implementation of policies and protocols, on a national scale, as part of the clinical governance agenda. Clinical governance is primarily concerned with effective audit and quality assurance systems that enable service provision to be monitored against local and national standards (DoH 2000a). Audit and quality assurance should be visible at every stage of the cancer journey, from diagnosis through to recovery or palliative care and death. Audit and research of cancer services are encouraged from a local trust level, through to a national level, in order to inform the development of new and existing services. One such national example is the NHS Cancer Patients' Survey for 1999–2000 (Airey et al. 2002), a survey that reports baseline data against *The NHS Cancer Plan* (DoH 2000a) and takes into account a number of aspects of care, including:

- location of care
- access to care
- the diagnosis
- tests and treatment
- communication and understanding
- involvement in care
- coordination and continuity of care
- symptom control
- discharge procedures
- the hospital environment
- outpatient appointments
- demographic difference in patients' experiences.

Therapeutic research

Since the 1990s there has been a clear increase in focus on the application of research findings in health-care practice, in order to ensure the provision of an evidence-based health service (Sackett et al. 1996, Regan 1998, Upton, 1999). This is linked to the increasing drive for specialist higher education (Expert Advisory Group on Cancer 1995) that is accredited by a university. The emphasis is on maintaining up-to-date knowledge in relation to cancer nursing practices, while developing a core of transferable skills in health-care professionals working with people with cancer, which encourage and enable a climate of life-long learning. Such transferable skills include research awareness and critical analysis skills which enable the evidence to be appraised systematically (Sackett et al. 1996) and the application of research processes to contribute to the body of professional evidence (Regan 1998, Upton 1999).

Despite the emphasis on the development of transferable skills through higher education to enable evidence-based practice, Mead (2000) proposes that the implementation of research findings into health-care practice remains highly complex. Attempts to integrate research findings into practice may prove fruitless unless the key staff members involved are included as major stakeholders and allowed to have ownership of the change. Traditionally it is accepted that change is most powerful when it comes from the 'bottom up' rather than being imposed from above (Iles and Sutherland 2001); however, the current emphasis in cancer services, as in other areas of the health service, is predominantly government led, focusing on the achievement of standards and targets. This government drive provides further impetus for change, for the benefit of service users, and also enables the allocation of appropriate resources to support change and development in order that services are ultimately improved.

Since the publication of *The Calman–Hine Report* (Expert Advisory Group on Cancer 1995), a number of strategic changes have been implemented from a central level in order to improve cancer services. The first major change was the reconfiguration of cancer services nationally to resolve the observed inequities in outcomes across the country. This resulted in the development of coordinated systems of care from primary care trusts, through cancer units in district general hospitals providing care and treatment for people with commonly occurring cancers, to cancer centres providing specialist care for common and less common cancers, in addition to specialist diagnostic and therapeutic techniques such as radiotherapy. A subsequent key development has been the cancer networks (DoH 2000a), of which there are currently 34 in the UK (see earlier).

Cancer networks are supported in their work by the Cancer Services Collaborative (CSC). The CSC offers an improvement partnership in a nationally funded NHS programme designed to make improvements in the way that cancer services are delivered to patients, through the NHS Modernisation Agency (DoH 2003a) and reflecting the improvement targets set out in *The NHS Cancer Plan* (DoH 2000a). Fundamental to the changes is an emphasis on collaborative working between service managers and the whole multidisciplinary team. The CSC is committed to supporting local clinical teams to explore and redevelop their own systems of working, in line with good change management practice (Iles and Sutherland 2001) so that:

- there is certainty and choice for patients
- care is preplanned and prescheduled at times to suit patients
- unnecessary delays to and restrictions on access are removed
- the patient and carer experience is improved through the provision of a personalized, consistent service
- the best care is provided, in the best place, by the best person/team (DoH 2003a).

The CSC improvement programme is a three-phase programme that started in 1999, with 9 pilot networks and 51 projects. It was expanded successfully to phase II in April 2001 to encompass all 34 cancer networks across England. Phases I and II focused on improvements in key cancers including cancers of the breast, bowel, lung, gynaecological, urological and upper gastrointestinal. Each project team produces a monthly report of progress against locally agreed priorities, which help to deliver the National Cancer Plan target (DoH 2000a). As a result, a series of 'service improvement guides' has been published by the CSC which share some of the practical improvements implemented by clinical teams and detail how they were achieved (see www.modern.nhs.uk/cancer). The third and final phase of the CSC improvement partnership started in April 2003. The intention of phase III is to make service improvement part of everyday business and activity in order to ensure the following:

- Patients and carers remain at the centre of redesigning processes so that their views form the basis of service improvement.
- Service improvement is integrated and sustained to provide long-term benefits, building on the work done in breast, lung, gynaecological, urological and colorectal cancers (NHS Executive 1997a).
- Service improvement work is aligned to ensure that it meets the local priorities identified by clinical teams, the cancer networks, strategic health authorities and primary care, through local delivery plans.
- Teams are supported to use the collaborative methodology to improve the services that they deliver (DoH 2003a).

The CSC focuses its work not only on specific tumour sites, but also on core service areas such as patient and carer experience, endoscopy, radiology, chemotherapy, radiotherapy and primary care (DoH 2003a). A large number of projects are taking place in each of these areas, with targets and definitions set by the teams involved. As well as enabling the developments of standards and guidelines for cancer care services, the project teams, in collaboration with the CSC, disseminate their work through professional development events. Resources developed by the project teams and the CSC, such as the chemotherapy toolkit, are available on the CSC website (www.modern.nhs.uk/cancer).

Notably, the work of the CSC has resulted in the publication of a *Manual of Cancer Services Assessment Standards* (DoH 2001d), which has served as a basis for national audit and the development of local, regional and national action plans in cancer care services (DoH 2001c, Richardson et al. 2002). *The Nursing Contribution to Cancer Care* (DoH 2000b) proposes that the nursing involvement in cancer care services is vital at every stage of the patient's cancer journey, with skilled and knowledgeable staff offering appropriate and timely support both to patients and to those around them who are affected by the cancer diagnosis. The nursing contribution is led by senior oncology nurses at local, regional and national levels, who are actively practising cancer care and also involved in the strategic development of the cancer nursing workforce through service planning and operational management, education, research and policy-making. This work requires a clear commitment to collaborative working with other colleagues in the NHS, with key stakeholders in the voluntary services, professional organizations and professional regulatory bodies, as well as a commitment to political activity and action in support of cancer care services (DoH 2001c). The nursing contribution is therefore evident in all the cancer service developments since 1995, from local to national levels, through individual and local teamwork to collaborative work with the cancer networks and the CSC, through research and the development of policies and protocols for care delivery.

One such example is the work of the Cancer Nursing Advisory Group (DoH 2003b), established in 2002 and that undertook work until July 2003, to address the action plan required to implement *The NHS Cancer Plan* (DoH 2000a) and *The Nursing Contribution to Cancer Care* (DoH 2000b). The key areas of work resulted in guidelines for practice in relation to the patient pathway and a managed career pathway in cancer care. A systematic review also led to the development and publication of a new competency framework for cancer nursing by a working party of cancer nurses from around England. The competency framework is based on behavioural rather than task-oriented competencies, and includes knowledge/skills/aptitude competencies, aligned to four categories: the health-care support worker, registered practitioner, senior registered practitioner and consultant practitioner (DoH 2003b), which reflects those used in *The Nursing Contribution to Cancer Care* (DoH 2000b). The framework is designed to reflect the competencies required by all nurses involved in the provision of care to cancer patients and not just those who are cancer specialists. The competency framework covers five key themes:

1. Cancer patient journey: understanding cancer, health promotion and education, screening, the treatment process.
2. Supportive care: interpersonal skills, informing, involving and supporting patients, patient education and training, rehabilitation and survivorship, meeting the palliative care needs of cancer patients, fertility and sexuality.
3. Multiprofessional and organizational team working.
4. Self: leadership, self-management and professional accountability.
5. Organization: managing resources, research and practice development, political policy awareness, inequalities in care, succession planning and governance.

In addition to policy development, *The Calman–Hine Report* (Expert Advisory Group on Cancer 1995) and *The NHS Cancer Plan* (DoH 2000a) support the development of new knowledge for cancer care services through a wide range of research that explores every aspect and stage of the cancer journey from a range of professional perspectives. Thus, professional knowledge informs practice in relation to the patient experience through nursing research, as well as in relation to treatment outcomes through therapeutic research.

In relation to colorectal cancer, the term therapeutic research refers largely to the medically driven research that provides an evaluation of the outcomes of medical interventions and therapies. This research often takes place as part of large multicentre clinical trials which compare and evaluate the efficacy of new therapies or surgical techniques against existing ones, or which evaluate alternative methods and modes of administration of existing proven therapies. These research projects are led by oncology clinicians, who are commonly supported by a wider team of professionals, including research nurses who work with a patient caseload, administer research therapies and collect data in a key coordinating role.

Therapeutic research takes place in three phases. Phase 1 research is usually associated with brand-new treatments. The research occurs in carefully controlled experimental conditions on a range of people with different cancers, where the intention is to establish the response rate in different situations as well as the general toxicity profile. At this stage the results of the treatment may be largely unknown, so patients participating in the studies are fully informed that this is highly experimental and may not ultimately benefit their own care. Phase 2 research studies usually take place in highly controlled experimental conditions where there is a high level of clinical support available for the patient. Phase 2 studies enable greater analysis of the effect of the treatment on specific cancers, and the patient population is therefore selected according to their cancer and disease stage, as informed by the initial findings of the phase 1 studies. Phase 3 studies are undertaken in cancer centres and cancer units across the country, using care facilities and services available to the population. The final phase normally consists of a comparison of the new treatment with existing treatments or a new treatment delivery mode with existing modes. Data are collected throughout phase 3 of the study, to inform research bodies, health-care professionals and national quality groups responsible for commissioning cancer care services which treatment is the most effective.

The emphasis on developing new research studies and evaluating practices is high. At the same time, each study possesses unique characteristics and features, so it is impossible to summarize the current research here. However, a comprehensive list of some of the latest colorectal research projects can be found on the Cancer Research UK website (www.cancerresearchuk.org). The cancer networks provide a central forum for review and appraisal of the research evidence (NHS Executive 1997b). Responsibility for dissemination of best practice (NHS Executive 1997a, National Cancer Guidance Steering Group 2004), including the development of policies and protocols, lies with the cancer networks.

It is clear that nursing staff in cancer care services have a responsibility to progress knowledge for the benefit of cancer service users, either through direct involvement in the research process or by critical appraisal and dissemination of relevant work. The reality is that many nursing staff, working in an increasingly acute environment, have little time to undertake primary or secondary research, even if highly motivated. In addition, Regan (1998) proposed that many nurses are put off reading and implementing research because of its perceived irrelevance to practice in general and the academic language used. The increasing focus on continuing professional development and the completion of formal courses to support specialist knowledge development means that there is a reducing problem in relation to nurses who lack the necessary skills to undertake a critical appraisal of the evidence and present a case of need (Connolly and O'Neill 1999, Upton 1999). A poor appraisal of the research evidence could result in a change in practice that does not improve patient care or clinical outcomes. As such, it is proposed that there should be formal mechanisms available whereby health-care staff can get advice and assistance with the above, which might include formal support from clinical governance departments within health-care trusts (Waters 1997, Regan 1998, Simpson et al. 1999).

Education

Central recommendations for the development of cancer services (Expert Advisory Group on Cancer 1995, DoH 2000a, 2000b) act as an authority for cancer care professionals to undertake formal educational development and, in so doing, they are supported to develop skills for life-long learning and working, including the research process, strategies and approaches for the management of change. Thus, higher education institutions and practitioners work in collaboration in order ultimately to improve services for the patient and those close to them who are affected by the cancer diagnosis.

Conclusion

Cancer care provides a clear focus of activity for service development and improvement, led centrally by government initiatives and policies but also concentrating on support for service audit and development at a local level, led by health-care professionals working at the coal face, in collaboration with managers, voluntary services, professional organizations and professional regulatory bodies. The increasing emphasis on the dissemination and implementation of best practices, informed by a critical appraisal of the research, requires a clear emphasis on the individual and team development of core skills to support this work. The emphasis, through access to higher education and continuing professional development programmes, is on the development of critical appraisal and questioning skills as part of the drive towards developing skills to support self-motivated life-long learning. In addition the need to be politically engaged and committed to the improvement of cancer care services for the benefit of the patient is of the utmost importance, both through the knowledge, awareness and dissemination of key initiatives and through active involvement in service audit and improvement to support central initiatives.

Summary of key points

- Colorectal cancer is one type of cancer that has received specific attention in terms of the improvement of cancer care services.
- Subsequent to the publication of the Policy Framework for Commissioning Cancer Services, a number of policy and guidance documents have been published, under the guidance of a National Cancer Director to guide the further development of cancer services, including cancer networks and cancer services collaboratives.
- The main driver and function of these structures are to continue to streamline cancer services and to develop local, regional and national policies, based on the best available evidence, in order to maximize the outcomes of cancer care and treatment through a skilled and committed workforce.

- Audit and research of cancer services is encouraged from a local trust level, through to a national level, in order to inform the development of new and existing services. Service improvement work is aligned to ensure that it meets the local priorities identified by clinical teams, the cancer networks, strategic health authorities and primary care, through local delivery plans.
- It is clear that nursing staff in cancer care services have a responsibility to progress knowledge for the benefit of cancer service users, either through direct involvement in the research process or by critical appraisal and dissemination of relevant work.

References

Airey C, Becher H, Erens B, Fuller E (2002) National Survey of NHS Patients – Cancer: National overview 1999/2000. London: HMSO.

Boyle P (1998) Some recent developments in the epidemiology of colorectal cancer. In: Bleiberg H, Rougier P, Wilke H-J (eds), Management of Colorectal Cancer. London: Martin Dunitz.

Cancer Research UK (2003a) Cancerstats: Incidence – UK factsheet. April 2003. London: Cancer Research UK.

Cancer Research UK (2003b) Cancerstats: Mortality – UK factsheet. February 2003. London: Cancer Research UK.

Connolly M, O'Neill J (1999) Teaching a research based approach to the management of breathlessness in patients with lung cancer. European Journal of Cancer Care 8: 30–6.

Department of Health (1999) A National Service Framework for Mental Health. London: HMSO.

Department of Health (2000a) The NHS Cancer Plan: A plan for investment, A plan for reform. London: HMSO.

Department of Health (2000b) The Nursing Contribution to Cancer Care. London: HMSO.

Department of Health (2001a) Diabetes National Service Framework. London: HMSO.

Department of Health (2001b) Older People's National Service Framework. London: HMSO.

Department of Health (2001c) The NHS Cancer Plan – Making Progress. London: HMSO.

Department of Health (2001d) Manual of Cancer Services Standards. London: HMSO.

Department of Health (2002) Cancer: National overview 1999/2000. London: HMSO.

Department of Health (2003a) Cancer Services Collaborative: Improvement partnership. A Quick Guide. London: HMSO.

Department of Health (2003b) Cancer Nursing Advisory Group. London: HMSO (available from www.doh.gov.uk).

Dunlop M (1997) Science, medicine, and the future: colorectal cancer. British Medical Journal 314: 1882–5.

Expert Advisory Group on Cancer (1995) The Calman–Hine Report: A policy framework for commissioning cancer services. London: HMSO.

Iles V, Sutherland K (2001) Organisational Change: A review for health care managers, professionals and researchers. London: London School of Hygiene and Tropical Medicine.

Mead P (2000) Clinical guidelines: promoting clinical effectiveness or a professional minefield? Journal of Advanced Nursing 31(1): 110–16.

National Cancer Guidance Steering Group (2004) Improving Outcomes in Colorectal Cancer, Updated manual. London: National Institute for Clinical Effectiveness.

NHS Executive (1997a) Improving Outcomes in Colorectal Cancer. London: HMSO.

NHS Executive (1997b) Improving Outcomes in Colorectal Cancer: The research evidence. London: HMSO.

NHS Executive (2000) Improving the Quality of Cancer Services (Health Service Circular). HSC 2000/021. London: HMSO.

Regan J (1998) Will current clinical effectiveness initiatives encourage and facilitate practitioners to use evidence-based practice for the benefit of their clients? Journal of Clinical Nursing 7: 244-50.

Richardson A, Miller M, Potter H (2002) Developing, Delivering and Evaluating Cancer Nursing Services: Building the evidence base. London: HMSO.

Sackett D, Rosenberg W, Muir Gray J et al. (1996) Evidence-based medicine: what it is and what it isn't. British Medical Journal 312: 71-2.

Simpson L, Madhok R, Whitty P (1999) Collecting, maintaining and using evidence of clinical effectiveness: experience at a district health authority. Health Library Review 16: 43-69.

Tattersall MHN, Thomas H (1999) Recent advances: oncology. British Medical Journal 318: 445-8.

Upton D (1999) Attitudes towards, and knowledge of clinical effectiveness in nurses, midwives and health visitors. Journal of Advanced Nursing 29: 885-93.

Waters EA (1997) Improving clinical effectiveness: a practical approach. Journal of Evaluation of Clinical Practice 3: 255-64.

Chapter 5

Bowel cancer surgical management

Barbara Stuchfield

Despite increased awareness, improved screening and surgery techniques, bowel cancer remains the second leading cause of death in women, following breast cancer, and the third in men, after lung and prostate cancer (Cancer Research UK 2003) (see Chapters 2 and 3).

In 1998 there were approximately 10 000 deaths from colon cancer and 6000 from rectal cancer. Five per cent of patients will have a synchronous tumour, i.e. more than one primary at the same time; 5% with one primary will have another at some time in the future (metachronous tumours) (Keighley and Williams 1999b). About 25% of colorectal cancer occur in the right side and transverse colon, 40% are sited on the left transverse and in the sigmoid colon, and 35% in the upper and lower rectum and anus (Keighley and Williams 1999b) (see Chapter 3).

The diagnosis of colon or rectal cancer is devastating news to most individuals, especially those with little information about the disease. Patients and family members may have to adapt to long-term changes in the individual's health status and reduction in income as well as, in some instances, to a poor prognosis. The fear of the cancer recurring may always be present in the patient's mind (see Chapter 9).

Based on the recommendations of *The Calman–Hine Report* (Expert Advisory Group on Cancer 1995) and the NHS Executive (1997a, 1997b), 'gold standard' guidelines were introduced to ensure equity of treatment and high-quality care for the improvement of the overall outcomes and mortality rate in colorectal cancer.

Diagnosis and staging

The initial assessment must include a thorough medical history, abdominal examination and a simple digital examination. This may be followed by flexible sigmoidoscopy, colonoscopy or a barium enema to visualize the whole colon. Biopsies of abnormal tissue may be taken at this time for histological confirmation. The biopsy results confirm diagnosis and if positive further investigations will be undertaken to stage the extent of the disease. See Chapter 3 for more detail.

After this the multidisciplinary team (MDT) make a treatment plan.

Management of colon cancer

The management of colorectal cancer has a multi-prong approach, and may include surgery, with resection and anastomosis to restore intestinal continuity as the primary treatment for early stage cancer (Finnegan 2000), and adjuvant therapies such as postoperative radiotherapy and chemotherapy. The treatment may be one option or a combination of all three modalities.

Curative surgery involves the complete excision of the primary tumour, ensuring that the margins around are tumour free, preferably 2–5 cm from the tumour to prevent local recurrence (Williams 1996). The resection of adjacent structures may be necessary provided that the associated vascular pedicle and the complete lymphatic clearance to the drainage area of the tumour can be safely excised (Keighley and Williams 1999b).

Unfortunately, about 50% of patients will either have metastatic disease discovered at surgery or will later have recurrence of the disease (Lederman 1997).

A palliative procedure involves limited excision of the tumour, bypass of the cancer, laser treatment, stenting (Harris et al. 2001, Bhardway and Parker 2003) or a defunctioning procedure, e.g. a stoma. A combination of chemotherapy and radiation may be prescribed if a radical surgical procedure is not possible; each of these is designed to alleviate the patient's symptoms.

Surgical management of liver metastases can be successful, but must be performed by an experienced hepatic surgeon.

Bowel cancer

The overwhelming majority of large bowel cancers are adenocarcinomas, between 5 and 20% of all polyps showing either a cancer or cancer *in situ* after the pathological results (Keighley and Williams 1999b).

High-risk groups

Ulcerative colitis

Patients with a long history, 10 years or more of ulcerative colitis involving the whole colon, are at greater risk of developing bowel cancer (see Chapter 3). They should be offered regular colonoscopic surveillance. If premalignant changes are found, surgery is recommended and entails removal of the colon and rectum, and formation of an end-ileostomy.

A restorative procedure to avoid a permanent stoma may be possible in patients with dysplastic changes or early cancer and in multifocal disease, as long as local clearance can be achieved (Keighley and Williams 1999b).

Preoperative preparation

Preoperative counselling is essential if the patient is to be psychologically prepared to cope with a variable functional outcome (Salter 1988), and should be undertaken by a nurse specialist or experienced person who has a sound knowledge base of colorectal cancer and the disease process (see Chapter 9).

Preoperative management

Colorectal cancer surgery is performed under general anaesthetic, so every effort must be made to improve or control other medical conditions such as cardiac or respiratory disease. Anti-thrombosis prophylaxis, such as subcutaneous Clexane and compression stockings, must also be used appropriately.

Many surgeons will prescribe a bowel preparation regimen using either stimulant or osmotic laxatives for 1–2 days before surgery to reduce the risk of faecal contamination at surgery. This may cause some dehydration and replacement of fluid loss is essential. Sometimes patients cannot tolerate large volumes of water, squash or black tea, and intravenous fluid may be necessary. A low-residue diet may be allowed up until the day before surgery, but some surgeons prefer a fluid-only regimen after laxative ingestion.

Broad-spectrum antibiotics, including protection against anaerobic organisms during surgery, are usually prescribed.

Where surgery will involve the formation of a stoma, the stoma care nurse or an appropriately trained nurse assesses the potential location on the abdomen (see Stoma siting, page 78).

Postoperative care

Postoperative management varies between surgeons and many units have standard protocols for the perioperative care of each patient. Generally the patient is allowed to drink water as soon as gastrointestinal function is established. Food is not introduced for several days. During this time the intravenous route maintains the fluid balance. The urinary catheter is removed when the urinary output is satisfactory and monitoring is no longer required.

Epidural or patient-controlled analgesia may be used immediately after surgery and reduced to oral pain control when appropriate. Caution should be used giving medication rectally if the patient has undergone low rectal anastomosis because it may cause a perforation.

Drains are removed when the output has significantly decreased, and clips/sutures are removed usually on the tenth postoperative day. Discharge is organized once bowel function has become fully established, although patients must be advised that bowel action and control may be erratic for several weeks after surgery.

If a stoma has been raised the stoma nurse specialist will help the patient with the practical care and offer appropriate psychological support.

Surgery for colon cancer

The surgical management of colon and rectal cancer have to be considered independently of each other, because there are standard procedures for the treatment of colon cancer and few other options, whereas the treatment of rectal cancer is multifaceted, needing many considerations.

Cancer of the right colon

Right hemicolectomy (Figure 5.1)

Through a midline incision, a laparotomy is performed to allow the colon to be resected. The caecum, ascending colon, hepatic flexure and proximal half of the transverse colon, and 5–10 cm of the terminal ileum, are mobilized and retracted towards the midline; the peritoneal reflection along the right paracolic gutter is divided. Any small blood vessels in the peritoneum are electrocoagulated before cutting. The blood supply to this segment includes the mesentery, together with the ileocolic, right colic and the right branch of the middle colic artery.

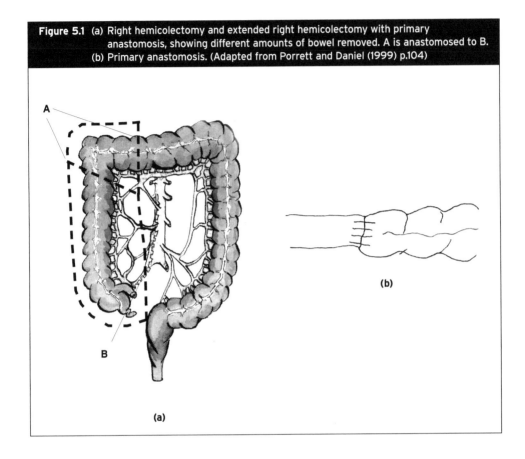

Figure 5.1 (a) Right hemicolectomy and extended right hemicolectomy with primary anastomosis, showing different amounts of bowel removed. A is anastomosed to B. (b) Primary anastomosis. (Adapted from Porrett and Daniel (1999) p.104)

These arteries are divided and ligated. The transverse colon is divided by transversely stapling its distal side or alternatively it is divided between crushing clamps. Similarly the ileum is divided between crushing clamps. The associated lymph nodes and lymphatics are removed with the colon from the retroperitoneum and omentum, and an anastomosis is performed as either an end-to-side (end of ileum to side of transverse colon) or end-to-end anastomosis, using sutures or a staple cutter.

If the tumour adheres to the surrounding structures, these are removed en bloc with the tumour during the operation, without entering any malignant tissue.

Extended right hemicolectomy (Figure 5.1)

This requires a more radical operation when the length of the resection is increased, leaving only the distal third of the transverse colon for anastomosis. This more radical procedure ensures that the entire lymph drainage from the right colon is included in the resection.

Cancer of the left colon

Left hemicolectomy (Figure 5.2)

This operation is performed for all tumours of the descending and sigmoid colon. Surgery entails removing colon from the transverse section, up to and below the sigmoid colon. The peritoneal reflection on the lateral side of the colon is divided; the blood supply includes the left branch of the middle colic artery, the left colic artery and the superior haemorrhoidal artery. These are removed together with the lymph nodes. The mid-transverse colon is clamped and divided. Similarly, the sigmoid colon is clamped. The divided transverse colon is then anastomosed to the upper rectum.

A defunctioning stoma may be required to protect the anastomosis; therefore patients need to be counselled preoperatively. Assessment by the colorectal nurse specialist (CNS) is essential whenever there is a possibility of stoma formation.

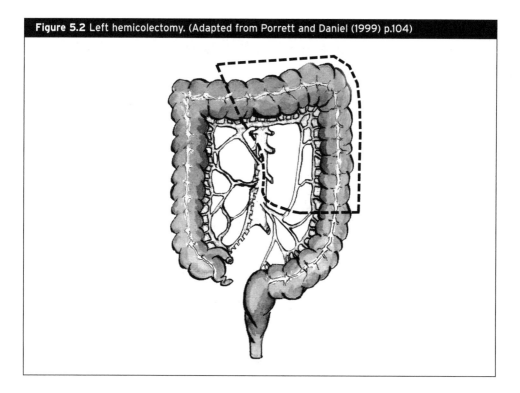

Figure 5.2 Left hemicolectomy. (Adapted from Porrett and Daniel (1999) p.104)

Cancer of the transverse colon

Transverse colectomy

Tumours of the transverse colon are rare; the surgery performed depends on the co-morbidities of the patient, exact site of tumour and anatomical variation of the blood supply of this area. Nowadays, an extended right hemicolectomy is usually preferred for all tumours as far distal as the splenic flexure. However, transverse or extended left hemicolectomy with removal of the transverse colon is performed under some circumstances.

Cancer of the sigmoid colon

Sigmoid colectomy (Figure 5.3)

Cancer of the sigmoid can be removed by a less extensive procedure than a radical left hemicolectomy. The technique is similar; the sigmoid colon is removed but only the sigmoid vessels are divided from the inferior mesenteric artery. This ensures a good blood supply to most of the left colon, which is then anastomosed to the upper rectum at the level of the sacral promontory.

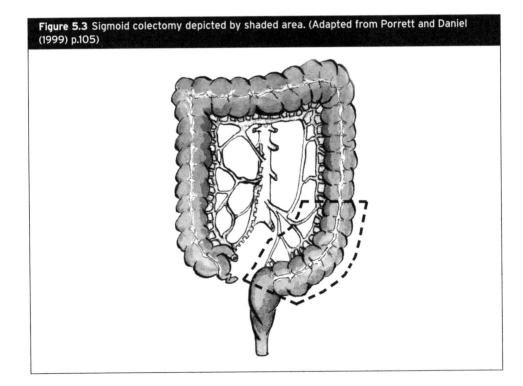

Figure 5.3 Sigmoid colectomy depicted by shaded area. (Adapted from Porrett and Daniel (1999) p.105)

Restorative proctocolectomy (ileal-anal pouch)

This technique (Figure 5.4) was developed in 1978 by Sir Alan Parks (Parks and Nicholls 1978) to restore gastrointestinal function after removal of the colon and rectum. It is a recognized procedure now used extensively for patients with ulcerative colitis and familial adenomatous polyposis (FAP).

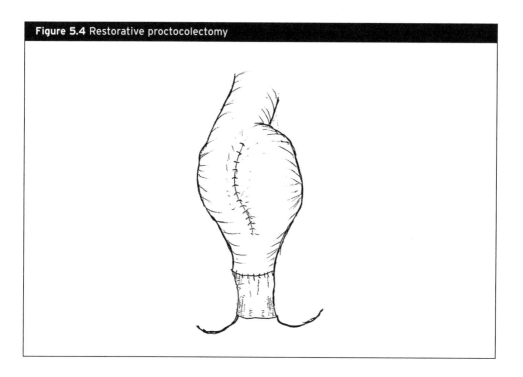

Figure 5.4 Restorative proctocolectomy

In some specialist units this procedure is used for patients who have developed dysplastic changes in their bowel or multifocal cancers from ulcerative colitis. The operation is an alternative to a permanent stoma; it is a complex procedure performed in one, two or three stages, depending on the patient's physical condition, nutritional state and immunosuppressant therapy such as steroids, which may have been part of the treatment regimen for ulcerative colitis.

Subsequent bowel function, and any potential problems such as pouchitis and possible incontinence, should be discussed in depth during the preoperative preparation (see Further reading).

A standard proctocolectomy is performed in which the entire large bowel and rectum are removed. This technique uses up to 50 cm of small bowel, which is constructed to form a faecal reservoir; although there are many configurations of pouches, the most common appear to be in the 'J', 'S' or 'W' shape. The 'J' design is the simplest and the most widely used reconstruction, it distends, has good capacity and empties readily (Nicholls 1993).

An ileal–anal anastomosis joins the pouch to the anal canal. The lower rectum lining (mucosectomy) is stripped, in order to reduce any likelihood of recurrent ulcerative colitis, and subsequent cancer or adenomatous disease (Fazio et al. 1993). Either a hand-sewn or a stapled anastomosis is performed and a covering ileostomy, which can be closed at a later date. In some instances a rectal tube can be inserted into the pouch to drain faecal fluid, thus avoiding a covering stoma; this is usually removed 7–10 days after surgery.

Hartmann's procedure (Figure 5.5)

Hartmann's procedure may be indicated for cancer of the rectosigmoid or an obstructing lesion. This operation may be performed for patients with diverticular disease or bowel perforation.

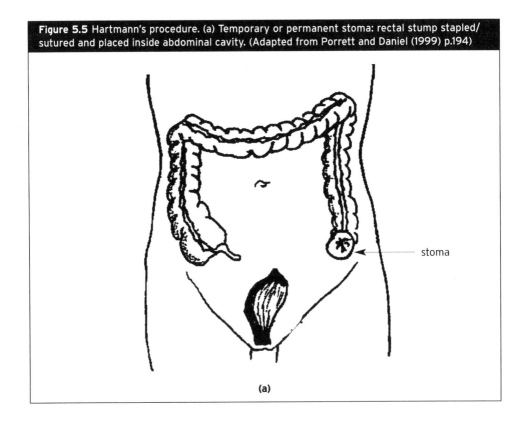

Figure 5.5 Hartmann's procedure. (a) Temporary or permanent stoma: rectal stump stapled/ sutured and placed inside abdominal cavity. (Adapted from Porrett and Daniel (1999) p.194)

stoma

(a)

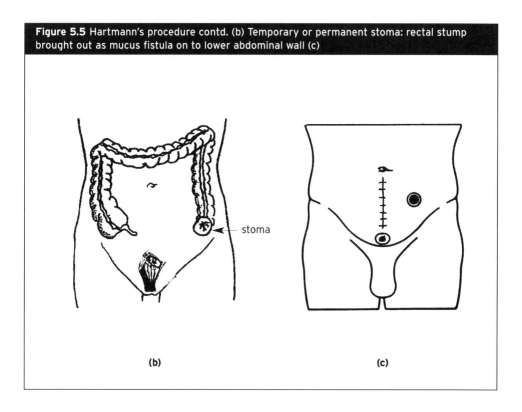

Figure 5.5 Hartmann's procedure contd. (b) Temporary or permanent stoma: rectal stump brought out as mucus fistula on to lower abdominal wall (c)

stoma

(b)　　　　　　　　　　(c)

A standard left hemicolectomy is performed as previously described with an end-colostomy fashioned at the time of surgery. The rectal stump can either be closed with a stapling instrument or manual suturing or brought out at the lower end of the abdominal incision line and termed a 'mucus fistula'. The mucus fistula or distal end is non-functional. Management problems as a result of position, 'flush stoma' and mucus leakage require the patient to wear a small ostomy pouch or appropriate dressing.

Closure of the stoma after Hartmann's procedure

This type of operation allows for stoma reversal and bowel anastomosis at some future stage, which entails connecting the sigmoid colon to the rectal stump. However, a third of these patients will never have their stoma closed. Surgical morbidity is as high as, and comparable to that of, the initial operation. Problems commonly associated with re-anastomosis are sepsis and, in the long term, stenosis at the connection site (Gregg 1987). Many patients manage to cope well with their stoma and do not wish to pursue further surgery.

Laparoscopy

There is a place for laparoscopic surgery in colorectal disease, but its use remains limited in most centres in the UK. It is often used as an integral part of an open procedure, or to raise a stoma.

Visualization of the internal organs is much clearer via a laparoscope, but the inability to palpate other organs and the difficulty of organ retrieval is a controversial topic among surgeons. Iatrogenic injuries to the ureters and major vessels, the inability to identify the colonic lesion and removal of the wrong segment of bowel have been reported from the USA (Wexner et al. 1993).

A critical issue after laparoscopic surgery for cancer is the problem of recurrence of tumour at the port site, not only the site through which the specimen is delivered, but all port sites (Wexner and Cohen 1995).

If this technique is offered, it must be by a trained team of specialists for best possible outcomes with full audit (Salum et al. 1999).

Postoperative complications

Anastomotic leak

Although patients undergoing colectomy may suffer any of the complications associated with major abdominal surgery, such as a chest or wound infection, anastomotic breakdown is a major source of morbidity. The overall significant leak rate after resection of a colonic tumour is currently in the region of 4% (Mella et al. 1997). The incidence for colonic surgery is lower than that after low rectal stapled anastomosis, where the leak rate may range from 3 to 18% (Keighley and Williams 1999b).

Anastomotic leak may present in a variety of ways; onset may be gradual, with warning signs such as a pyrexia, tachycardia and abdominal distension resulting from a paralytic ileus.

In the patient with localized peritonitis whose condition remains stable, a conservative approach with systemic antibiotics may be appropriate; however, should a patient develop sudden generalized peritonitis and septicaemic shock, resulting from rapid faecal contamination of the peritoneal cavity, surgery will be urgently required and a stoma is usually raised to divert the faecal stream. Unfortunately the mortality rate from faecal peritonitis is high at over 50% (Keighley and Williams 1999b, Phillips 2001).

Intestinal obstruction

Twenty per cent of all surgery for colorectal cancer will present as an emergency, and 16% will present with intestinal obstruction (Mella et al. 1997).

Large bowel obstruction is a dangerous condition carrying an overall mortality of 16.5% and management demands a high level of expertise (National Cancer Guidance Steering Group or NCGSG 2004). The mortality rate from subsequent bowel perforation intensifies with age and with widespread disease, giving a figure of 26% and increasing to 69% in those aged over 70 years (Parker and Baines 1996).

Intestinal obstruction may cause abdominal pain, distension, nausea and vomiting, which can be faecal in appearance. The main cause of an obstructing lesion is cancer, although adhesions from previous surgery or a diverticular mass cannot be excluded.

Generally patients with an incompetent ileocaecal valve can be managed conservatively using a nasogastric tube and intravenous therapy. Surgery may be indicated after diagnostic radiographs, and computed tomography (CT) of the abdomen, to remove a section of bowel or to bypass the obstruction. A stoma may be raised proximal to the obstruction.

In some centres it is now standard practice to treat patients with left-sided malignant large bowel obstruction, above the lower third of the rectum, with self-expanding metal stents (SEMSs). These may provide adequate palliation of the obstructed bowel, while radiotherapy or chemotherapy treatment is given (Cole et al. 2000; see Chapters 6 and 7).

Stoma surgery

Surgical developments in large bowel cancers over the past few decades have tended to reduce the number of permanent stomas constructed. Currently the trend is to perform a temporary stoma wherever possible with a view to closure at a later date.

A stoma is an artificial opening in the bowel, which can be temporary or permanent. A permanent stoma is carried out when there is no prospect of re-joining the colon to restore bowel continuity.

Reasons for stoma formation

- Where the disease requires removal of the anal sphincter mechanism such as a low rectal cancer and in specific incidents of anal cancer.
- Where distal pathology indicates a defunctioning stoma such as perforation or protection of the distal anastomosis site after surgery or during intensive radiotherapy or combined chemoradiotherapy.

Stoma siting

Preoperatively, the patient is sited for a stoma by the colorectal nurse specialist (CNS) for stoma care, or an experienced nurse, to ensure that the stoma is positioned correctly on the abdomen. A poorly sited stoma may cause leakage problems and delay rehabilitation. Assessment must consider, among other things, the patient's mental and physical attitude, and ethnicity. Ideally an informed and participating patient can assist in this process (see Further reading).

The located site should lie within the rectus abdominis sheath, on a flat part of the abdomen away from previous scars, creases and skinfolds. It is important to involve the patient in all the stages of this process, encouraging the patient to adopt various positions, i.e. bending, sitting and standing. This will enable the optimal site to be selected (McCahon 1999, Elcoat 2003).

Patients should have the opportunity to wear an appropriate pouch under their usual style clothing to ensure that the pouch is not visible above the waistline; this may not be possible when trousers or skirts are worn at too low a level.

Disabled people, of whatever sort and/or if wheelchair dependent, require specific consideration. Stoma siting will need to reflect and accommodate their individual circumstances, such as sitting in the wheelchair or lying in bed (Elcoat 2003, Borwell and Breckman 2004).

Patients should be able to see the proposed stoma mark to facilitate the practical aspects of stoma care management, such as the correct application of an ostomy pouch. Sites (Figure 5.6) should be clearly marked with a permanent ink pen and covered with an adherent clear dressing to prevent the mark fading or inadvertently transferring to another site when the patient bends. In some instances, both sides are marked, when surgeons are undecided about the type of stoma required, i.e. a colostomy or ileostomy (see Further reading).

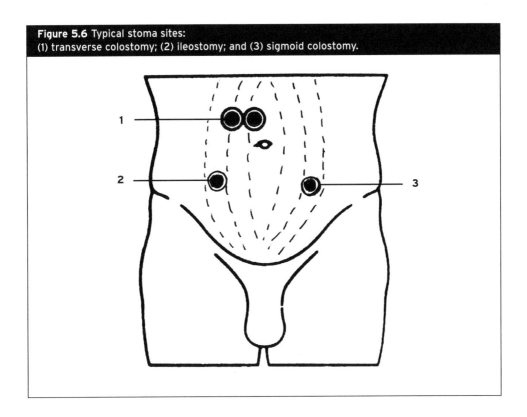

Figure 5.6 Typical stoma sites:
(1) transverse colostomy; (2) ileostomy; and (3) sigmoid colostomy.

Considerations for stoma siting

Areas to avoid:

- Proposed incision line
- Hipbones
- Previous operation scars, bulges, creases
- Under pendulous breast
- Waistline
- Current skin condition, e.g. psoriasis
- Position of straps/corsets that could occlude the area, e.g. prosthetic limb, surgical appliances and proximity of existing stoma.

Life after stoma surgery may present difficulties. Specialist nurse intervention is vital because they are equipped with the appropriate expertise to cope with most problems, whether practical or emotional (see Chapters 8 and 9).

Stoma surgery

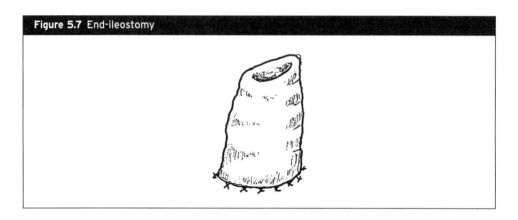

Figure 5.7 End-ileostomy

End-ileostomy (Figure 5.7)

An end-ileostomy is usually sited through the right rectus sheath or muscle. This site is used to reduce the risk of a parastomal hernia occurring later on in life. The distal end of the ileum is separated using a staple cutter or by dividing the bowel between clamps. About 5 cm of terminal ileum is then exteriorized through the abdominal wall at a site previously marked.

The bowel is opened once the clamps are removed or the staple line excised, and the stoma is everted to form a spout, ideally between 3 and 5 cm to aid stoma management and minimize effluent leakage. Mucocutaneous absorbable sutures are used to secure the ileal wall to the subcutaneous tissues around the stoma (see Chapter 9).

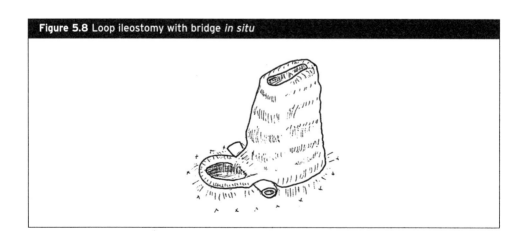

Figure 5.8 Loop ileostomy with bridge *in situ*

Loop ileostomy (Figure 5.8)

A loop ileostomy can be constructed without a full laparotomy, delivered directly through the abdominal wall via a trephine or laparoscopically.

A trephine is made as described previously. The rectus sheath is opened and the terminal ileum identified. A loop of intestine is delivered through the abdominal wall. An enterostomy (opening) is made in the distal limb and the proximal lip everted. Mucocutaneous dissolvable sutures are placed to secure the stoma to the skin surface. A plastic rod may be placed beneath the bowel at the junction of the ileum and skin to support the bowel; the proximal limb is everted and sutured as described for the end-ileostomy.

The CNS or experienced ward nurse will generally remove the rod after 5–10 days dependent on the individual surgeon's instructions.

End-colostomy (Figure 5.9)

An end-colostomy is usually placed in the left iliac fossa, although this may vary depending on the type of operation performed. The stoma is constructed through the rectus sheath, and the colon is divided using a staple

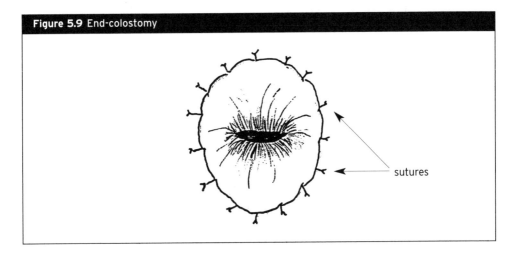

Figure 5.9 End-colostomy

sutures

cutter or separated between two clamps. A trephine is sited and the colon delivered through the abdominal wall. It is sutured as described above.

Loop colostomy (Figure 5.10)

A loop colostomy may be sited right, left or transverse. Construction is the same as for a loop ileostomy.

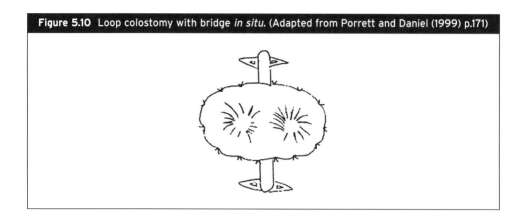

Figure 5.10 Loop colostomy with bridge *in situ*. (Adapted from Porrett and Daniel (1999) p.171)

A transverse loop colostomy is usually placed in the right upper quadrant of the abdomen, above the patient's waistline, and can cause problems with clothing and management technique.

Double-barrelled colostomy (Figure 5.11)

Two sections of the descending or sigmoid colon are brought out on to the abdomen through an incision in the left iliac fossa. The two lengths of bowel are sutured together and everted as previously described for loop ileostomy.

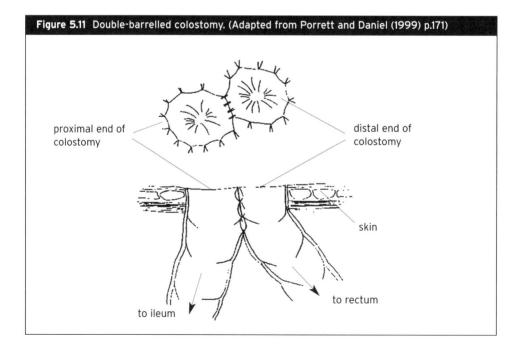

Figure 5.11 Double-barrelled colostomy. (Adapted from Porrett and Daniel (1999) p.171)

Divided colostomy (Figure 5.12)

This procedure is performed to avoid any contamination of the defunctional section of bowel. The affected area of bowel is resected and a colostomy is formed from the proximal end. The distal end of bowel (non-functional) is secured on to the abdominal wall separated by a bridge of skin to develop a divided colostomy.

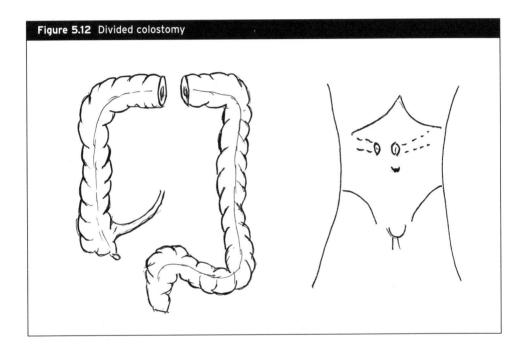

Figure 5.12 Divided colostomy

Surgery to the rectum

Cancer of the rectum is treatable and often curable when localized. Surgery is the primary treatment and curative in about 50% of all patients (Keighley and Williams 1999b). Prognosis is related to the degree of cancer infiltration through the bowel wall and lymph node involvement.

The surgical management of rectal cancer is more complex than that of colonic cancer. A decision has to be made whether the anal sphincters can be preserved or removed; this is determined by the distance of the cancer from the anal margins. Currently, rectal tumours with 2-cm clearance from the dentate line can be managed by sphincter-saving techniques (Keighley and Williams 1999a).

Over the past three decades the trend has moved away from abdomino-perineal excision to sphincter-saving procedures. Improved surgical techniques and the use of stapling devices, to access difficult areas, are mainly responsible for these changes.

Quality of life issues, such as preservation of continence, reasonable bowel frequency, and the avoidance of permanent sexual and urinary dys-function, should also be a decision-making consideration when performing sphincter-saving techniques.

Abdominoperineal excision of the rectum (Figure 5.13)

Abdominoperineal excision of the rectum (APER) was the 'gold standard' procedure for cancer of the rectum for decades, but now the proportion of rectal tumours treated in this way has reduced by two-thirds since 1985 (Keighley and Williams 1999b). This technique may, however, be performed for:

- cancers within 5 cm of anal margin
- cancer of the anus, which has not responded to chemotherapy or radiotherapy
- effective surgical clearance achievable only by complete rectal excision.

Preoperative radiotherapy or chemotherapy may be necessary to shrink the tumour size to aid surgical removal (see Chapters 6 and 7).

Preoperative counselling by the CNS or appropriate team member is vital when a permanent end-colostomy is indicated, with the significant

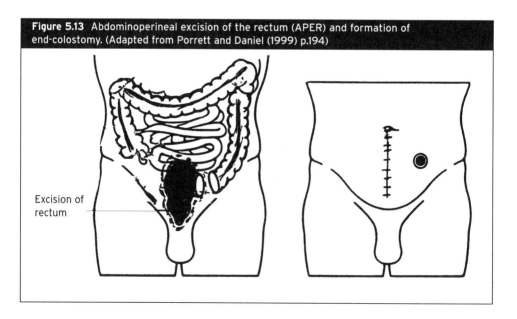

Figure 5.13 Abdominoperineal excision of the rectum (APER) and formation of end-colostomy. (Adapted from Porrett and Daniel (1999) p.194)

Excision of rectum

risk of sexual impairment and/or urinary dysfunction. The procedure entails removal of the sigmoid colon, rectum, sphincter mechanism and anus using a coordinated approach.

Two surgeons are necessary for this combined operation. One surgeon will undertake an abdominal approach to perform a sigmoid colectomy in the standard way (previously described) with an end-colostomy. The second surgeon, adopting a perineal approach, removes the rectum and sphincter mechanism.

Perineal approach

The anus is closed with a heavy suture to prevent faecal soiling; an incision is made in the perineum, around the anal verge.

Using cautery the fat is incised circumferentially around the anus to where the level of the anal coccygeal ligament is reached posteriorly. Cautery is used to incise the levator muscles and the rectum is further dissected and freed posteriorly and laterally.

The specimen is passed down by the abdominal operator and removed through the perineum.

High anterior resection (Figure 5.14)

The operation of choice for cancer of the upper third of the rectum, 12 cm above the anal verge, is anterior resection. During this operation the sigmoid colon and part of the rectum are removed. The bowel is dissected to

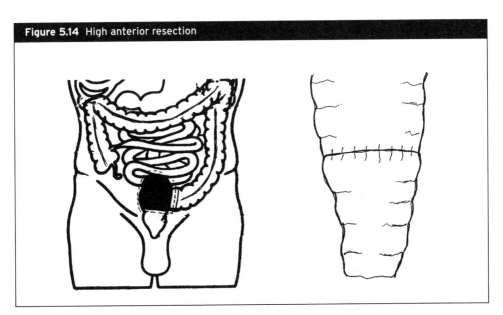

Figure 5.14 High anterior resection

5 cm below the tumour and cut between crushing clamps. An anastomosis is formed between the descending colon and any remaining rectum.

Low anterior resection (Figure 5.15)

The sigmoid colon and entire rectum are removed. The descending colon is anastomosed to the anal canal, about 5–6 cm from the anal verge. This technique allows complete removal of the mesorectum, leaving a small amount of rectum sufficient to attain an end-to-end anastomosis, using a stapling device. Where possible the autonomic nerves are preserved to protect sexual function, providing that all evidence of tumour can be safely removed.

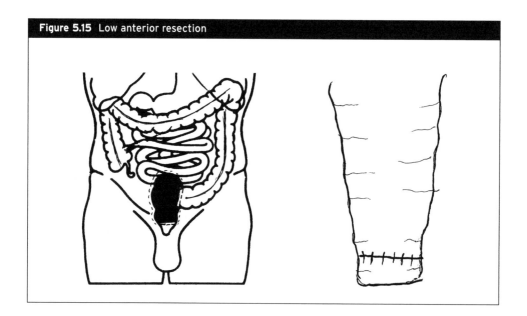

Figure 5.15 Low anterior resection

Surgery to remove the mesorectum at the time of operation is now favoured by many surgeons to reduce the incidence of local recurrence (Heald et al. 1982, Steele 1999).

There may be local recurrence because of inadequate local excision, or if the primary tumour was disrupted at the time of the surgery. Malignant cells may implant themselves into the tumour bed, port site, wound or at the anastomosis (Phillips et al. 1984).

There is an increased risk of anastomotic breakdown after low anterior resection, occurring in 10–20% of patients, so all patients undergoing surgery should be prepared for a temporary stoma (Mella et al. 1997).

Disturbed anorectal function may occur after anterior resection (anterior resection syndrome); this is related to the level of the anastomosis from the anal verge, i.e. the lower the anastomosis, the greater the risk, combined with impaired capacity of the neorectum and reduced anal pressures (Keighley and Williams 1999).

Symptoms may include urgency of defecation, frequency, incontinence to flatus and faeces; subsequent perianal excoriation may occur as a result. These problems may improve over several months. In the meantime diarrhoea can be managed in a variety of ways; anti-diarrhoeal medicines, e.g. loperamide, and dietary advice may help. Perianal excoriation may require some emollient cream, e.g. Sudocream.

If life has been severely affected by continence problems the patient may opt to have a permanent stoma.

Formation of colonic pouch (Figure 5.16)

An end-to-end coloanal anastomosis operation may have poor functional results (Parc et al. 1986), and as a consequence there is a move towards construction of a colonic pouch at the time of surgery. This type of pouch is able to store faeces and improve urgency of defecation and continence problems.

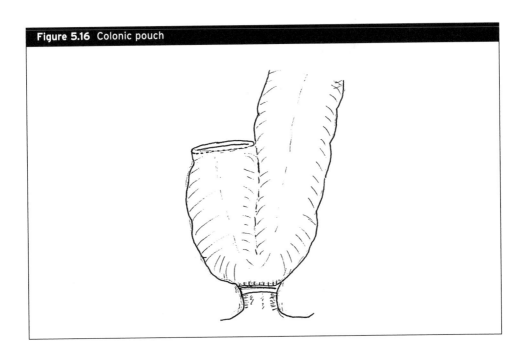

Figure 5.16 Colonic pouch

In this operation the entire sigmoid colon and rectum are removed and a 5-cm-long colonic pouch is constructed. An anastomosis is made between the colonic pouch and anal canal, which may either be hand sewn or stapled.

Local treatment of cancer

A snare (wire loop) can remove small adenomatous polyps during an endoscopic procedure; the histopathology results will determine if there is complete excision. If the polyp is too large for local removal, or where the excision has been incomplete, more extensive surgery may be required.

Conventional local excision can be performed via the transanal (Buess et al. 1985) or trans-sphincter approach for removal of early small tumours. This technique is less invasive and may be advantageous in elderly patients or those with co-morbidity, such as heart failure. A laparotomy may have to be undertaken if the histopathology results show that the margins of resection were not tumour free.

Surveillance and follow-up

Most patients, after surgery, are currently followed up in colorectal clinics. Annual colonoscopy surveillance is arranged yearly for 4–5 years to detect any new cancers (metachronous), together with liver ultrasonography and carcinoembryonic antigen (CEA) measurement to detect metastases (see Chapter 3).

Electrically stimulated neoanal sphincter

This is an innovative technique, performed within some specialist units in the UK. For some patients the concept of having a permanent stoma is so repugnant that they ask for reconstructive surgery. This technique, pioneered at the Royal London Hospital in the UK (Mander et al. 1996) and in Maastricht in the Netherlands (Baaten et al. 1995), is performed in several stages over a period of time, usually 12 months, in patients whose rectum has been removed or plans were made for rectal excision of the cancer.

This operation involves the reconstruction of a neoanal sphincter by using the gracilis muscle from the inner thigh. An abdominal excision of the rectum is performed. The colon is brought down and a coloperineal anastomosis performed in the original position of the anus. The gracilis muscle is then transposed and wrapped in a gamma configuration (Figure 5.17) around the 'anus' to create a new sphincter: it is finally sutured to the bone of the ischial tuberosity.

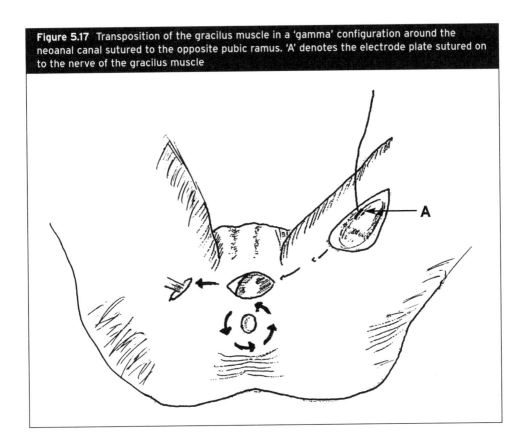

Figure 5.17 Transposition of the gracilus muscle in a 'gamma' configuration around the neoanal canal sutured to the opposite pubic ramus. 'A' denotes the electrode plate sutured on to the nerve of the gracilus muscle

A small electrode plate is placed on the nerve of the gracilis muscle; wires are tunnelled to the in-planted stimulator (similar to a cardiac pacemaker), which is sited in the anterior abdominal wall. The gracilis muscle is a fatigable muscle and unable to sustain continuous contractions. To enable continuous contractions to be maintained, thus occluding the anal canal, a non-fatiguable muscle is required. The implanted stimulator achieves this.

A remote control device is used to program the stimulator, by transmitting radio waves through the patient's skin. This device allows the voltage and stimulation frequency to be modified and adjusted to the level of contraction within the muscle tension of the anus. An external remote device allows the patient to operate the stimulator's on/off switch, to control defecation (Figure 5.18).

Detailed preoperative counselling and information about this complex procedure, including potential loss of functional outcomes and other associated complications, are vital (Abercrombie et al. 1996, Eccersley et al. 1997).

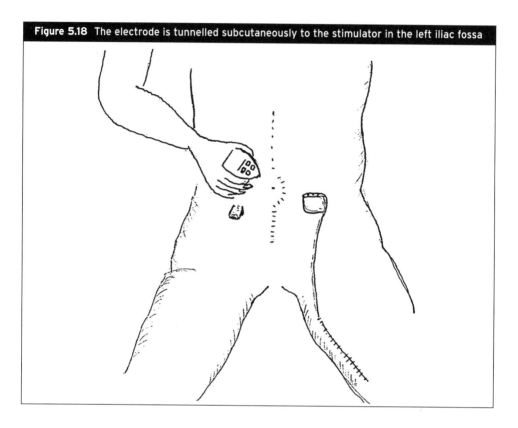

Figure 5.18 The electrode is tunnelled subcutaneously to the stimulator in the left iliac fossa

Stool evacuation may be difficult after this operation, but there are some devised management strategies to assist with these problems.

Anal cancers

Cancer of the anal margin and canal are rare, accounting for 4% of all large bowel cancers; however, there is some evidence that the incidence is increasing (Scholefield 2001). This is because infection with the human immunodeficiency virus (HIV) in gay communities in the USA is rising (Wexner et al. 1987).

Of anal cancers 80% are squamous in origin, and arise from the squamous epithelium of the anal margin and anal canal (Keighley and Williams 1999b). Symptoms may include bleeding, pain, a lump and pruritis ani.

Treatment of this condition is usually a combination of chemotherapy and radiotherapy, although radical surgery such as an APER may be required for resistant disease. Patients with anal cancer should be managed by specialist MDTs (NCGSG 2004).

Human papillomavirus

Immunological factors such as HIV are thought to play an important role in the malignant potential of this virus-induced cancer. A weakened immune system, e.g. following renal transplantation, becomes unable to fight infections and viruses, such as the human papillomavirus (HPV) type 16 or 18; these may become more active and trigger the development of squamous cell cancer.

Intraepithelial neoplasia

Anal intraepithelial neoplasia (AIN) is a relatively benign condition; however, for a high-grade AIN (III) there is a potential risk of cancer. Small lesions can be locally excised; a larger excision may require a skin graft to cover the area excised, with a temporary stoma raised to promote wound healing.

Adenocarcinoma of the anal canal is usually a very low rectal cancer that has spread downwards to involve the canal; true adenocarcinomas do occur, arising from the anal glands, and pass rapidly outwards into the sphincter muscles. The tumour may respond well to radiotherapy but should still be treated with radical surgery such as an APER and a permanent colostomy.

Conclusion

Despite greater awareness of bowel cancer symptoms many people are reluctant to seek medical help. Less than 50% discuss bowel problems with their doctor because of embarrassment and fear (Johnson and Lafferty 1961).

Using MDTs with members who are experts in bowel cancer, the planned, individualized patient-focused care may achieve the 'gold standard' practice advocated by *The Calman–Hine Report* (Expert Advisory Group on Cancer 1995) to decrease mortality rates in the UK.

Summary of key points

- Recognize the signs and symptoms of bowel cancer.
- Understand the relevance of screening and staging process in the surgical management of bowel cancer.
- Relate the location of cancer to the type of operation performed and the rationale for stoma formation.
- Increased awareness of sphincter-conserving techniques and other morbidities, e.g. sexual dysfunction.
- The importance of preoperative counselling and support.
- Understanding the surgical management of bowel cancer to enable the nurse to provide essential and relevant information.

Acknowledgement

Thanks to Miss S Clark, FRCS, Colorectal Surgeon, St Bartholomew's and the Royal London Hospital for her support.

References

Abercrombie JF, Rogers JR, Williams NS (1996) Total anorectal reconstruction results in complete anorectal reconstruction. British Journal of Surgery 83: 57-9.
Baaten CGMI, Geerdes BP, Adang E et al. (1995) Anal dynamic graciloplasty in the treatment of intractable faecal incontinence. New England Journal of Medicine 332: 1600-5.
Beart RW Jr, Van Heerdon JA, Beahrs OH (1978) Evolution in the pathological staging of carcinoma of the colon. Surgery, Gynaecology and Obstetrics 146: 257.
Bhardway R, Parker MC (2003) Palliative therapy of colorectal cancer: stent or surgery? Colorectal Diseases 5: 518-21.
Borwell B, Breckman B (2004) Bowel stomas how and why they are created. In: Beckman B (ed.), Stoma Care, 2nd edn. London: Elsevier, in press.
Buess G, Theiss R, Gunter M (1985) Endoscopic surgery to the rectum. Endoscopy 17: 31-5.
Cancer Research UK (2003) Colorectal cancer fact sheet. London: Office of National Statistics (www.cancerresearchuk.org/stastics).
Cole SJ, Boorman P, Osman H et al. (2000) Endoluminal stenting for relief of colonic obstruction is safe and effective. Colorectal Disease 5: 282-7.
Eccersley AJP, Maw A, Williams NS (1997) Quality of life can be improved by anorectal reconstruction. International Journal of Colorectal Disease 12: 130.
Elcoat C (2003) Stoma Care Nursing. Birmingham: Hollister Ltd.
Expert Advisory Group on Cancer (1995) The Calman-Hine Report: A policy framework for commissioning cancer services. London: HMSO.
Fazio VW, Tjandra JJ, Lavery IC (1993) Techniques of pouch construction. In: Nicholls J, Bartolo D, Mortensen N (eds), Restorative Proctocolectomy. London: Blackwell Scientific, pp. 18-33.
Finnegan WC (ed.) (2000) Cancer from Diagnosis to Palliative Care. CD-ROM. London: Macmillan Cancer Relief/Centre for Medical Education, University of Dundee.

Gregg RO (1987) An ideal operation for diverticular of the colon. American Journal of Surgery 153: 285-90.

Harris J, Senagore AJ, Lavery IC et al. (2001) The management of neoplastic colorectal obstruction with endoluminal stenting. American Journal of Surgery 181: 499-506.

Heald RJ, Husband EM, Rya RD (1982) The mesorectum in rectal cancer surgery: the clue to pelvic recurrence. British Journal of Surgery 69: 613-16.

Johnson JF, Lafferty J (1961) Epidemiology of faecal incontinence. The silent affliction. American Journal of Gastroenterology 91: 33-6.

Keighley RB, Williams NS (eds) (1999a) Surgery of the Anus, Colon and Rectum, 2nd edn. London: WB Saunders.

Keighley RB, Williams NS (1999b) Surgery for colorectal cancer. In: Diseases of the Anus, Colon and Rectum. London: WB Saunders, pp. 1062-118.

Lederman J (1997) Funding Issues in the Treatment of Cancer. London: Royal College of Physicians.

McCahon S (1999) Faecal stomas. In: Daniels N, Porrett T (eds), Essential Coloproctology for Nurses. London: Whurr Publishers.

Mander BJ, Abercrombie JF, George BD et al. (1996) The electrically stimulated gracilis neosphincter as part of total anorectal reconstruction after abdominoperineal excision of the rectum. Annals of Surgery 224: 702-11.

Mella J, Biffin A, Radcliffe AG et al. (1997) Population based audit of colorectal management in two UK health regions. British Journal of Surgery 84: 1731-6.

National Cancer Guidance Steering Group (2004) Improving Outcomes in Colorectal Cancer, Updated manual. London: NICE.

NHS Executive (1997a) Improving Outcomes in Colorectal Cancer. Guidance on commissioning cancer services. London: Department of Health.

NHS Executive (1997b) Improving Outcomes in Colorectal Cancer: The research evidence. London: Department of Health.

Nicholls RJ (ed.) (1993) Restorative Proctocolectomy, Vol. 5. Oxford: Blackwell Scientific, pp. 53-82.

Parc R, Tiret E, Frileux P et al. (1986) Resection and coloanal anastomosis, for rectal carcinoma. British Journal of Surgery 73: 139-41.

Parker MC, Baines MJ (1996) Intestinal obstruction in the patient with advanced malignant disease. British Journal of Surgery 83: 1-2.

Parks AG, Nicholls RJ (1978) Proctocolectomy without ileostomy for ulcerative colitis. British Medical Journal ii: 85-8.

Phillips RKS (ed.) (2001) Rectal cancer. In: Colorectal Surgery, 2nd edn. London: WB Saunders, pp. 90-105.

Phillips RKS, Hittenger R, Biesousky L et al. (1984) Local recurrence after 'curative surgery' for lower bowel cancer: the overall picture. British Journal of Surgery 71: 12-16.

Porrett T, Daniel N (1999) Essential Coloproctology for Nurses. London: Whurr Publishers.

Salter M (1988) Altered Body Image: The nurse's role. London: Scutari Press.

Salum MR, Wexner SD, Daniels N et al. (1999) Laparoscopic colorectal surgery In: Porrett T, Daniels N (eds), Essential Coloproctology for Nurses. London: Whurr Publishers.

Scholefield JH (2001) Anal cancer. In: Phillips RKS (ed.), Colorectal Surgery, 2nd edn. London: WB Saunders, pp. 125-37.

Steele RJC (1999) Anterior resection with total mesorectal excision. Journal of the Royal College of Surgeons, Edinburgh 44: 40-5.

Wexner SD, Cohen SM (1995) Port site metastases after laparoscopic surgery for cure of malignancy: a plea for caution. British Journal of Surgery 82: 295-8.

Wexner S, Milsom J, Dailey T et al. (1987) The demographics of anal cancer are changing. Identification of a high-risk population. Diseases of the Colon and Rectum 30: 942-6.

Wexner SD, Johansen OB, Nogueras JJ et al. (1993) Laparoscopic colorectal surgery: a prospective assessment and current perspective. British Journal of Surgery 80: 1602-5.

Williams NS (ed.) (1996) Colorectal Cancer. New York: Churchill Livingstone.

Further reading

Black P (2000) Holistic Stoma Care. London: Baillière Tindall in association with the Royal College of Nursing.

Keighley MR, Pemberton JH, Fazio VW et al. (eds) (1996) Atlas of Colorectal Surgery. New York: Churchill Livingstone.

Keighley RB, Williams NS (eds) (1999) Surgery of the Anus, Colon and Rectum, 2nd edn. London: WB Saunders.

Mortensen N, Madden MV (1993) Pouchitis – acute inflammation in pouchitis. In: Nicholls RJ, Bartolo D, Mortensen N (eds), Restorative Proctocolectomy. London: Blackwell Scientific, Chapter 8.

Phillips R (ed.) (1999) Colorectal Surgery, 2nd edn. London: WB Saunders.

Stuchfield B (1997) The electrically stimulated neoanal sphincter and colonic conduit. British Journal of Nursing 6: 219–24.

Weiss EG, Johnson TE (1999) Colorectal cancer. In: Porrett T, Daniel L (eds), Essential Coloproctology for Nurses. London: Whurr Publishers, pp. 97–116.

Educational resources

City University and St Bartholomew's School of Nursing and Midwifery (1999) An Interactive Guide to Stoma Care Nursing. CD-ROM. London.

Dansac Ltd. Principles of Stoma Siting. VHS cassette.

Elcoat C (2003) Stoma Care Nursing. CD-ROM. Wokingham: Hollister Ltd.

Chapter 6

Chemotherapy

Tanya Andrewes

Background

This chapter provides an overview of the principles of chemotherapy treatment in relation to cancer care in general, with specific reference to colorectal cancer. It enables the exploration of the effects of the five groups of chemotherapeutic agents and provides guidelines for nursing care based on the nursing process as a model for care.

The term 'chemotherapy' literally refers to 'drug therapy' in the widest context, i.e. any type of drug therapy used to treat disease. In the context of cancer care specifically it is more accurate to refer to 'cytotoxic chemotherapy', i.e. drug therapy that has the potential to kill cells.

Cytotoxic chemotherapy is just one of the key treatment modalities used in the care of people with cancer. Unlike surgery and radiotherapy that specifically enable localized treatment of cancer, chemotherapy and biological therapies have a systemic effect and thus have the potential to treat both local disease and disseminated metastatic disease. Cytotoxic chemotherapy works by interfering with the deoxyribonucleic acid (DNA) in the cells, damaging the genetic material so that the cell is unable to replicate itself. Although cytotoxic chemotherapy has the potential to inflict massive damage on the cell's genetic material and thus kill the cell, it also has the potential to work more subtly, creating just enough damage to activate the production of p53 and, in turn, the natural apoptosis (cell death) response (Weinberg 1998). Consequently, cancer cells that have lost their p53 production are seen to be more resistant to treatment because they are less likely to be encouraged into apoptosis.

Notably, because cytotoxic chemotherapy has a systemic action, its administration can also result in damage to healthy cells, potentially causing a considerable amount of toxicity, which is often best managed at specialist cancer centres and cancer units by skilled professionals (Souhami and Tobias 1998). An understanding of the background, actions and toxicities of cytotoxic chemotherapy is therefore vital for the provision of effective care and support to people with cancer and those closest to them who are affected by the cancer diagnosis.

Drug therapy for cancer was first discovered between 1940 and 1955, when it was observed that drugs such as nitrogen mustard (carmustine) actively shrink and kill cancer cells. When used alone cytotoxic chemotherapy is known as primary treatment. Since the initial discovery of its cytotoxic potential, chemotherapy has proved to be successful in curing a small number of cancers and improving survival when used as an adjunct or additional therapy to local control measures such as surgery. The purpose of adjuvant therapy is to kill microscopic cancer cells that may have begun to spread throughout the body and to ensure that the surgical margins are free of disease. Cytotoxic chemotherapy is increasingly given before other treatments such as surgery or radiation, in order to shrink the tumour and make it more amenable to intervention. This is known as neoadjuvant therapy. Cytotoxic chemotherapy is also used to provide effective palliation against the symptoms of advanced cancer (Holmes 1996).

Principles of chemotherapy treatment

Cytotoxic chemotherapy

Cytotoxic chemotherapy refers broadly to the use of drug therapies and of biological therapies (biotherapy) and immunological therapies (immunotherapy) – the increasing use of naturally occurring and synthetically manufactured substances to invoke a natural apoptosis response in the presence of cellular genetic abnormalities. Cytotoxic chemotherapy drugs exhibit their anti-tumour effects through their direct action on individual tumour cells. They ultimately cause cell death by altering the cellular DNA and preventing mitosis, or by initiating the apoptotic response through the stimulation of p53 production. The drugs are classified according to their precise action on the cell cycle. Therefore they are considered to be drugs that are either cell cycle phase specific (CCPS) or cell cycle phase non-specific (CCPNS).

Cytotoxic chemotherapy drugs are further classified into five groups according to their biochemical action:

1. Alkylating agents: the primary action of alkylating agents is to form cross-linkages between the DNA strands. Examples include cyclophosphamide and busulfan (busulphan). This group of drugs is CCPNS.
2. Antimetabolites: these work by blocking the enzymes necessary for synthesis of DNA. Examples include 5-fluorouracil (5FU), used in the treatment of colorectal cancer, and fludarabine. The antimetabolites are CCPS, exerting influence during the S phase.

3. Anti-tumour antibiotics: this group of drugs primarily interfere with DNA function but may also alter the cell membrane. Examples include bleomycin and epirubicin. They are CCPNS drugs.
4. Vinca alkaloids and plant derivatives: these drugs interfere with DNA replication by binding DNA strands together, so that they are unable to replicate. Examples include etoposide and vincristine. The vinca alkaloids and plant derivatives are CCPNS.
5. Miscellaneous agents: this group of agents is CCPNS, working in a range of ways to cause breaks and cross-linkages in the DNA strands in order to inhibit replication. Examples include irinotecan, a drug used in the treatment of colorectal cancer (see page 101).

Cytotoxic drugs are presented in a variety of forms for clinical use, including; intravenous, oral, intramuscular, intra-arterial, intravesical (directly into a vessel such as the portal venous system, delivered in the perioperative period to treat liver metastases) and topical application. The delivery mode is dependent on the cytotoxic drug and the cancer type and site. Apart from topical chemotherapy applied locally for skin cancer, cytotoxic chemotherapy is blood borne and thus has the potential to treat both primary disease and distant metastases. It therefore has utility in a variety of clinical settings from acute through to palliative care. Treatment for colorectal cancer is predominantly delivered intravenously.

Cell cycle specificity is highly relevant in terms of therapy. As CCPS drugs are active only at a particular point in the cell cycle whereas CCPNS drugs are active at any point in the cycle, this has implications for the drug regimen and delivery pattern used, e.g. 5FU, a common cytotoxic agent used in the treatment of colorectal cancer, has a CCPS action, so it exerts maximum effect during the S phase of the cell cycle. The S phase is the stage at which DNA synthesis and replication take place and this stage lasts for around 10–20 hours. As the cell cycle process is dynamic not all cells go through the same phase of the cell cycle at the same time, so if 5FU is administered intravenously over a short period of time it will affect only a small number of cells in the S phase at the time of administration. Furthermore, 5FU has a short half-life of around 20 min, which means that each 20 min the amount of drug available for use is halved. In the past, cytotoxic chemotherapy drugs such as 5FU would be delivered at a higher dosage in order to maximize the potential for action leading to cell death; however, knowledge about cell cycle specificity and observations in relation to dose-related toxicity led to the development of new delivery regimens. When administered continuously at a lower therapeutic dose, an increased level of cell death can be achieved through sustained contact of 5FU with cells at the S phase. Notably, the lower therapeutic dose enabled by this mode of delivery minimizes the actual and potential toxicities of the treatment. 5FU may be delivered continuously for either

12 or 24 weeks, with the dose titrated against the presence of diarrhoea and palmar/plantar syndrome, which are the main toxicities of this treatment. The intravenous administration of 5FU requires the placing of a central venous access device for the duration of the treatment.

Although cytotoxic chemotherapy treatments may be administered as single agents, they may also be administered in combination with other agents. Even though cancer develops from one single cell, the genetic events that occur as the tumour grows and spreads throughout the body result in varied biological and clinical behaviour. Therefore, tumours within one patient can vary in terms of the antigens present on the cell surface, the chromosomal abnormalities that present and the response to cytotoxic chemotherapy, e.g. a tumour mass in the lung might respond to a particular cytotoxic chemotherapy treatment whereas a tumour in the liver does not (Markman 1997). This phenomenon provides a good rationale for the use of combination chemotherapy regimens. A single chemotherapy drug may prove to be effective in the treatment of a specific cancer, but only when it is administered at such a high dose that life-threatening toxicity results. Combination regimens are carefully selected to exploit the potential of different drugs that are effective against specific tumour tissue, and that have different actions at different points in the cell cycle. Although the result is greater damage to the tumour cell, there is minimization of toxicity because of the careful selection of drugs that have different toxic effects.

Cytotoxic chemotherapy is commonly administered on a regular (cyclical) basis (weekly or monthly) in order to exploit the natural healing process of healthy cells and thus reduce the overall potential for toxicity. Significantly these drugs are not able to discriminate between healthy cells and cancer cells so, when administered, both cell populations sustain a level of damage. It is clear that healthy cells are able to repair themselves more rapidly than tumour cells (Holmes 1996). Cyclical chemotherapy regimens are calculated so that the drugs are administered as soon as the healthy cell population has recovered, but before the tumour cell population has recovered, exploiting the potential of increased damage to the cancer cells, but minimizing the toxic effects on the healthy cell population. The timing of treatment cycles is absolutely crucial because cycles given too frequently will result in increased damage of the healthy cells, causing severe toxicity, and cycles given too infrequently enable the tumour tissue to recover and even progress.

There is increasing interest in the timing of chemotherapy administration. Many biological processes are more active at certain times of the day, e.g. metabolism is higher when there is daylight and lower when it is dark. The result is an alteration in the rate of chemotherapy metabolism and excretion. It is proposed that the administration of chemotherapy at specific times in the day might increase damage to the tumour but result in less toxicity (Holmes 1997). An example of this is 'chronotherapy', where chemotherapy is administered at a double dose overnight because cancer cells are active but healthy cells rest. Ongoing research will enable clinicians to evaluate whether this technique is more effective than the conventional cyclical or continuous infusional therapy.

Cytotoxic chemotherapy causes a range of toxicities as a result of its non-discriminatory action on rapidly dividing tissue. Notably, the systemic mode of administration of chemotherapy means that widespread toxicity is likely, as opposed to the local effects seen in other cancer treatments such as radiotherapy. Potential systemic effects are outlined in Table 6.1. It is not inevitable that people receiving cytotoxic chemotherapy treatment will experience all the potential toxicities to any level, as the presenting effects depend on a number of factors. These include the drug group, its toxicity profile, the treatment schedule and dose, the route of administration, the type of cancer and the susceptibility of the individual patient (Holmes 1996). Toxicities of cytotoxic chemotherapy may present directly at the time of treatment (acute); they may be short term, presenting around 3–7 days after treatment has been administered (subacute), or long term, presenting at least 1 week after treatment. Not every patient will experience all of the common toxicities represented in Table 6.1 because each drug has different actions and toxicities.

Table 6.1 Potential toxicities of cytotoxic chemotherapy treatment for colorectal cancer

System	Potential toxicity	Likely onset
Central nervous system	Malaise and lethargy	ST/LT
Digestive system	Altered taste and smell	ST/LT
	Mucositis/stomatitis	ST
	Nausea and vomiting	LT
	Anorexia	LT
	Diarrhoea	ST
Integumentary system	Palmar/plantar syndrome	ST
	Rashes	A or ST
	General urticaria	ST
Venous system	Hypersensitivity	A
	Anaphylaxis	A
	Pain at infusion site	A
	Extravasation	A
	Flushing along vein	A
	Flushing of body	A
	Urticaria at vein	A
	Inflammation	A
Bone marrow	Bone marrow depression (characterized by anaemia, neutropenia and thrombocytopenia)	ST

A, acute; ST, short term; LT, long term

Understanding of the nature of potential toxicities is crucial in terms of planning and delivering sound nursing care and support for the patient. It is crucial that patients and their families receive specific information about anticipated effects tailored to their individual treatment regimen.

Immunological therapies

Immunological and biological response modifier (BRM) therapies are recent additions to the therapeutic treatments against cancer, although these are not currently used in the treatment of colorectal cancer. BRM therapies, which arose after observations that spontaneous regressions of some cancers occurred after bacterial infection, are based on natural manipulation of the immune system in order to provoke an apoptotic response. This is quite different to the action of chemotherapy which tends to attack the cancer cells directly.

Interferons, natural proteins that are formed when cells are exposed to a virus, activate macrophages, the immune cells that kill invading cells, and have anti-proliferative properties. The interleukins, protein cells that normally occur naturally within the body, activate neutrophils and lymphocytes and stimulate antibody production. Colony-stimulating factors increase the production of neutrophils and macrophages. Notably, the association between high dose and degree of response is not seen in BRM, where too high a dose will suppress the desired response (Markman 1997). The effects of BRM therapy may not become evident for several weeks or even months.

Chemotherapy for colorectal cancer

The mainstay of cytotoxic chemotherapy for both early and advanced stage colorectal cancer is 5FU (Moertel et al. 1990, Wolmark et al. 1993, Cancer Research UK 2003a). Administration is largely intravenous with cyclical regimens being the preference for early stage disease and continuous therapy for advanced disease. 5FU is commonly administered in combination with folinic acid, levamisole or leucovorin, agents that enhance its action and thus its effectiveness. Recently a tablet form of 5FU has been developed (capecitabine and Uftoral) and formally approved for use by the National Institute for Clinical Excellence (NICE) in the UK since May 2003, after clinical research (Cancer Research UK 2003a). The benefit of oral therapy, as opposed to intravenous therapy, is that the patient can administer the medication at home and therefore reduce the need for hospital visits and inpatient stays (Gerbrecht 2003). A central venous access device is not necessary, so the potential for compromising the body's immune system is reduced. In addition, the toxicity profile of the oral form of 5FU is less than that for the intravenous form. The toxicities for 5FU include diarrhoea, palmar/plantar syndrome, mucositis, nausea and pancytopenia, resulting in potential anaemia, increased risk of developing infection (neutropenia) and increased risk of bleeding (thrombocytopenia).

Irinotecan (CPT-11) is an intravenous cytotoxic chemotherapy drug that is used as a second-line treatment for colorectal cancer, when scans reveal that the disease has not responded to 5FU (Rougier et al. 1998). Administered as a cyclical regimen, it is likely to cause greater toxicity than 5FU, particularly an increased risk of intensified diarrhoea and a reduced white cell count (neutropenia), leading to an increased risk of infection. In addition, complete alopecia (hair loss) may occur with the administration of irinotecan (Cancer Research UK 2003a). A further cytotoxic chemotherapy drug was recently approved by NICE for colorectal cancer that has metastasized only to the liver. Oxaliplatin is used in conjunction with 5FU to reduce the size of liver metastases and facilitate removal by surgery (Cancer Research UK 2003a). The toxicities associated with the administration of oxaliplatin are mild, and usually consist of temporary neutropenia and tingling or numbness in the fingers and toes. This has implications for the patient with a stoma or a disability in relation to manual dexterity.

5-Fluorouracil is the treatment of choice for rectal cancer. Clinical trials have shown that intravenous 5FU acts as a radiosensitizer (Cancer Research UK 2003b), so it is often used in combination with radiotherapy (adjuvant therapy), in order to shrink rectal tumours and facilitate surgical removal of the diseased area as a result.

Patient assessment

Decisions about the clinical management of each patient are made collaboratively by the specialist colorectal cancer team, as advocated in the NHS guidelines (NHS Executive 1997a, 1997b, National Cancer Guidance Steering Group or NCGSG 2004). All decisions and the resultant treatment plan are documented in the patient's records in order to improve communications between members of the health-care team, in the endeavour to provide holistic care. The above factors, in addition to Dukes' classification of the tumour stage, are taken into account when planning cytotoxic chemotherapy treatment. Chemotherapy is usually indicated for Dukes' C and D colorectal cancer. Before the first treatment blood tests, radiographs or scans are performed in addition to a medical examination, in order to ascertain the suitability for specific cytotoxic chemotherapy drugs. If the chemotherapy drug to be used has a potential impact upon lung function, a lung function test will be performed before the start of therapy. Similarly, if the drugs selected for use have a potential impact on cardiovascular function, an ECG or echocardiogram may be performed. In addition to enabling assessment of health status and suitability for specific chemotherapy drugs, these tests often provide a baseline against which to measure progress throughout the duration of treatment. Regular blood tests will certainly be taken throughout the treatment in order to assess ongoing suitability for continued treatment and to guide dosing of the treatment or titration in the event of toxicity (Cancer Research UK 2003c).

The key to the effective nursing management of the person with cancer and his or her family, friends or carers is effective communication and in-depth holistic assessment. These factors enable the formulation of appropriate goals, negotiated between the nurse and the patient, and the planning of appropriate nursing interventions to meet the patient's needs. A useful framework for this purpose is the nursing process, a four-stage model to facilitate a coordinated approach to care, encompassing assessment, planning, intervention and evaluation. The nursing assessment of the person with cancer falls into four broad categories (psychological, physical condition and symptoms, knowledge about cancer and its treatment, and health surveillance/maintenance behaviours) that can be explored within the nursing process. In practice the nursing process is often used in conjunction with a formal theoretical nursing framework based on a particular philosophy and belief about the nature of nursing practice.

An example of a model used within oncology care is Roy's (1984) model for nursing, with adaptation as its focus and the role of the nurse to plan nursing interventions to resolve problems that prevent adaptation to a stimulus. Roy (1984) refers to stimuli that may either hinder or facilitate adaptation to current and future life circumstances. Roy (1984) advocates implementation of the model by first level assessment (identification of maladaptive behaviours), second level assessment (identification of stimuli), nursing diagnosis and establishment of goals in cooperation with the patient, supported by ongoing evaluation of behavioural outcomes and subsequent modification of nursing approaches. This reflects the nursing process and is based on the premise that quality of life will be improved if adaptation is facilitated. A key feature of the model is that underlying stimuli are identified from the start, so that intervention is aimed at the source of the problem rather than the symptoms, right from the beginning.

An alternative model used widely in the UK is the model of nursing of Roper et al. (1996). Their model is based on the philosophy that the patient's condition under normal circumstances, and his or her physiological/functional abilities should enable the patient to perform activities of daily living independently. This model encourages the nurse to consider the psychological, spiritual and socioeconomic impact of the patient's problems on lifestyle, although this aspect is less explicit and transparent, requiring skilled application of the model and creativity in practice. Again, the first level assessment is advocated in order to identify areas where the patient cannot independently manage activities of daily living, for whatever reason. The second level assessment enables the nurse to identify underlying problems or causes of dependence, so that appropriate nursing interventions can be planned, in collaboration with the patient.

Bredin et al. (1999) and Corner (1996) reinforced the importance of patients understanding their condition and coming to terms with it in relation to coping with their cancer diagnosis and its treatment. Therefore, it is essential that the patients and their carers have time to talk, to ask questions, and to express their fears and anxieties. Listening to each patient's personal story is essential in this context. Discussion and assessment enable the nursing staff to identify strategies already employed by patients to relieve the symptoms of their disease and/or the toxicities associated with their cancer treatment.

In the case of cancer, physical nursing care is largely focused on the proactive prevention of toxicity where possible and the prompt treatment of toxicity if it arises through planning appropriate nursing interventions. Therefore, a fundamental understanding of actual and potential toxicities, as described above, is crucial to effective care. Developments in care in terms of new approaches and therapies are ongoing and therefore it is impossible to provide a contemporary checklist of interventions for specific problems. Texts, such as that by Kaye (1994), provide an invaluable evidence-based resource to inform care planning and intervention. In addition to supporting patients through medical treatment to resolve chemotherapy toxicity, nursing staff should initiate a range of non-pharmacological and therapeutic nursing interventions, including the use of touch and comfort (Morse 1994) and education (Roberts et al. 1993). The nurse plays a crucial role in helping patients to come to terms with the condition and to develop coping strategies wherever possible. This care includes psychological support to help the patient come to terms with sexuality, relationship and work issues (see Chapters 8 and 9).

Chemotherapy drugs and related toxicities

In relation to the administration of cytotoxic chemotherapy treatment for colorectal cancer, and 5FU in particular, the common toxicities include gastrointestinal disturbance such as nausea and vomiting, a sore mouth, diarrhoea, palmar/plantar syndrome and altered bone marrow function.

Nausea and vomiting are frequently rated as the worst symptom of cancer and its treatment. There are very many factors implicated in its development and multiple causes are commonly identified in the individual patient with cancer. Chemotherapy is the primary cause. Chemotherapy drugs are recognized as foreign agents because they attack the body cells, so the natural response is to attempt to rid the body of the drugs. The phenomenon of nausea is commonly more distressing than the act of vomiting itself, which often provides some relief from the associated discomfort. Treatment depends on the cause and should take into account the inhibited absorption of oral medications, so alternative routes (intravenous/intramuscular/subcutaneous/rectal) should be used wherever possible.

Traditionally, chemotherapy-induced nausea and vomiting have been treated with dopamine receptor antagonists such as metoclopramide, which reduces gastric motility. Metoclopramide acts as a dopamine receptor antagonist at low doses and a serotonin $5HT_3$ antagonist at high doses. Its action is enhanced by the addition of the corticosteroid dexamethasone to the drug regimen. High-dose use of metoclopramide is limited and rarely used because of central nervous system side effects such as akathisia (the patient feels anxious and cannot sit still – dancing feet syndrome) and torticollis (contraction of the neck muscles). A preferable treatment is with $5HT_3$ antagonists, such as ondansetron in the first instance, providing good effect for around 48–72 hours after each course of acute treatment. Lorazepam is beneficial for the treatment of anticipatory nausea and vomiting associated with treatment. Many units implement evidence-based protocols for the management of nausea and vomiting (see Appendix, page 110). Additional measures include the following (Cancer Research UK 2003d):

- Avoiding eating or preparing food when feeling sick
- Avoiding fried foods, fatty foods or foods with a strong smell
- Eating cold or slightly warm food if the smell of cooked or cooking food causes nausea
- Eating several small meals and snacks each day
- Having a small meal a few hours before treatment
- Drinking lots of liquid, taking small sips slowly throughout the day

- Avoiding large amounts of liquid before eating
- Avoiding foods that irritate the mouth such as very salty or spicy foods, citrus fruits or rough foods such as toast
- Sucking fresh pineapple chunks to help to keep the mouth fresh and moist
- Using relaxation techniques to help reduce sickness
- Sipping ginger ale, taking herbal tablets or chewing crystallized ginger
- Wearing Seabands or having a course of acupuncture
- Avoiding too much activity around the time of chemotherapy treatment.

Mucositis is a common toxicity of 5FU treatment that can occur from 5 to 10 days after starting treatment (Cancer Research UK 2003e). The condition can be very painful and strong analgesia may be required, but with appropriate care the condition can resolve within 3–4 weeks. However, dose modification of the drug may be required to aid resolution. Good oral hygiene is essential to ensure that the mouth does not become infected, especially in the presence of pancytopenia. Additional measures to increase comfort include the following (Cancer Research UK 2003e):

- Avoid foods that taste strange
- Choose foods that have strong flavours (e.g. herbs, marinades and sauces) if all food tastes the same; note that ostomy patients should avoid spicy foods
- Clean the mouth and teeth gently every morning, evening and after each meal, using a soft-bristled or child's toothbrush
- Remove and clean dentures every morning, evening and after each meal
- If toothpaste stings, or brushing the teeth causes nausea, use a 'bicarbonate of soda' mouth wash instead
- Use dental floss daily but with care to avoid damaging the gums
- Keep lips moist by using Vaseline or a flavoured lip balm
- Avoid neat spirits, tobacco, hot spices, garlic, onion, vinegar and salty food when the mouth is sore
- Choose meals that are moist with gravies and sauces, to make swallowing easier
- Try to drink at least one and a half litres (3 pints) of fluid a day
- Report mouth ulcers to the doctor
- Suck fresh pineapple chunks to keep the mouth fresh and moist.

Diarrhoea is a condition that commonly manifests as a side effect of 5FU and irinotecan treatment or as a sign of gastrointestinal infection.

Infection should be ruled out before starting treatment with anti-diarrhoeal agents such as loperamide. Loperamide may be underused in the treatment of diarrhoea secondary to abdominal malignancy because of the fear of causing constipation (Kaye 1994). The use of skin moisturizers may provide relief of burning in the perianal area in the presence of profuse diarrhoea. The use of a bidet is advocated to maximize hygiene and comfort with gentle patting to dry the skin. Heightened awareness of this condition in patients with an ileostomy and giving contact details of the stoma care nurse are important because the visual appearance of an ulcerated, 'raw' stoma can be disturbing. Additional measures to increase comfort include (Cancer Research UK 2003e):

- Eating less fibre (raw fruits, fruit juice, cereals and vegetables)
- Drinking plenty of liquid to replace the fluid lost.

The ostomy patient may suffer additional problems as a result of diarrhoea. A review of the type of pouching system used is essential because a drainable pouch (if not usually worn) may need to be applied during the episode of diarrhoea, in order to reduce the number of pouch changes and thus prevent skin excoriation. Equally, the ileostomy patient could encounter electrolyte imbalance and dehydration.

The presence of any or all of the above symptoms (nausea and vomiting, diarrhoea, mucositis) normally necessitate referral to a dietitian for advice and monitoring (see Chapters 9 and 11).

Palmar/plantar syndrome is extreme soreness of the feet and hands, which can result in blistering and the feeling that the soles of the feet and the palms of the hand are burning up. It is a direct consequence of 5FU treatment and, although medication can be used to ease the problem, modification of the dose of the drug is essential to ensure resolution. Early identification and reporting of the problem are important to minimize potential or actual discomfort.

Chemotherapy drugs and radiotherapy treatment cause 'pancytopenia', which is a lowered total blood cell count, with characteristic production of immature cells from the bone marrow. Pancytopenia manifests as anaemia that causes dyspnoea and fatigue, thrombocytopenia, a low platelet count that renders the patient susceptible to spontaneous bruising and potentially life-threatening bleeding and neutropenia – a low white blood cell count that can potentially predispose to fatal septicaemia. Regular monitoring of the patient's blood count is therefore vital and additional precautions in relation to the control of infection and protection from trauma may be required to minimize the risks of bleeding.

Once the plan of care has been identified, documentation is crucial. This ensures that the care plan is clear to everyone involved in the delivery of that care and it ensures a baseline measure against which to evaluate the outcome of nursing actions. Regular evaluation and review are essential with adaptation of the care plan as required, to ensure the optimum benefits of care for the patient. Notably, clear and accurate documentation enables interventions and outcomes to be audited, so adding to the nursing contribution to clinical governance.

Safety considerations for staff handling cytotoxic chemotherapy drugs

Safety of health-care professionals who handle chemotherapy drugs is of the utmost importance. In addition to being very irritant, many cytotoxic chemotherapy drugs have the potential to induce mutagenic changes in an embryo or foetus, especially during the first trimester of pregnancy, or carcinogenic changes in healthy tissue. Nursing and medical staff who handle cytotoxic chemotherapy drugs do not ingest or absorb it directly, and therefore come into contact only with minuscule doses in comparison to the patients; however, it is believed that the effects of exposure are cumulative (Holmes 1996) and direct contact with chemotherapy drugs should be avoided. Most cytotoxic drugs are reconstituted in sterile preparation facilities within pharmacy departments, where health and safety procedures are in place and where risks to personnel handling the drugs are minimal. During cytotoxic chemotherapy administration practical protective measures that reflect universal precautions should be adopted to minimize the potential for direct contact with the drugs. This includes the routine use of protective clothing such as gloves and apron. As these drugs are commonly excreted by the kidneys body fluids should be treated as contaminated and universal precautions adopted when handling waste products. Equipment used for chemotherapy administration should be labelled as special waste and incinerated at high temperatures in accordance with the Control of Substances Hazardous to Health (COSHH) Regulations.

Nurses handling chemotherapy drugs on a regular basis should be screened annually for symptoms of exposure to chemotherapy, such as anaemia, neutropenia (reduced white blood cell count, particularly neutrophils) and thrombocytopenia. In addition urinalysis should be performed, enabling the occupational health department to monitor for mutagenic changes in the cells lining the bladder which are shed in the urine.

In conclusion, it is evident that cytotoxic chemotherapy treatments serve to help cure cancer in some cases, and to alleviate the effects of cancer in others. The use of chemotherapy drugs is complex and requires a sound understanding of the nature of the drugs, their actual and potential effects, and the health and safety issues relevant to their use. Research is ongoing and therefore it is essential to remain conversant with the latest recommendations, advice and developments in order to provide the highest standard of proactive and supportive nursing care.

Summary of key points

- Cytotoxic chemotherapy is just one of the key treatment modalities used in the care of people with cancer. It has a systemic effect and thus has the potential to treat both local disease and disseminated metastatic disease.
- Cytotoxic chemotherapy works by interfering with the DNA in the cells, damaging the genetic material so that the cell is unable to replicate itself.
- As cytotoxic chemotherapy has a systemic action, its administration can also result in damage to healthy cells, potentially causing a considerable amount of toxicity, which is often best managed at specialist cancer centres and cancer units by skilled professionals.
- Cytotoxic chemotherapy drugs exhibit their anti-tumour effects through their direct action on individual tumour cells. The drugs are classified into five groups, according to their precise action on the cell cycle.
- The delivery mode is dependent on the cytotoxic drug and the cancer type and site. Treatment for colorectal cancer is predominantly delivered intravenously.
- Cytotoxic chemotherapy causes a range of toxicities as a result of its non-discriminatory action on rapidly dividing tissue. Presenting effects are dependent on the drug group, its toxicity profile, the treatment schedule and dose, the route of administration, the type of cancer and the susceptibility of the individual patient.
- Toxicities of cytotoxic chemotherapy may present directly at the time of treatment (acute); they may be short term, presenting around 3-7 days after treatment has been administered (subacute), or long term, presenting at least 1 week after treatment. Understanding of the nature of potential toxicities is crucial in terms of planning and delivering sound nursing care and support for the patient.
- In relation to the administration of cytotoxic chemotherapy treatment for colorectal cancer, and 5FU in particular, the common toxicities include nausea and vomiting, a sore mouth, diarrhoea, palmar/plantar syndrome and altered bone marrow function.
- Nurses handling chemotherapy drugs on a regular basis should be screened annually for symptoms of exposure to chemotherapy, such as anaemia, neutropenia (reduced white blood cell count, particularly neutrophils) and thrombocytopenia.

References

Bredin M, Corner J, Krishnasamy M et al. (1999) Multicentre randomised controlled trial of nursing intervention for breathlessness in patients with lung cancer. British Medical Journal 318: 901-4.

Cancer Research UK (2003a) Chemotherapy drugs for bowel cancer. Updated 23 September 2003. Accessed from www.cancerresearchuk.org (18 November 2003).

Cancer Research UK (2003b) Chemotherapy with radiotherapy for bowel cancer. Updated 7 October 2003. Accessed from www.cancerresearchuk.org (18 November 2003).

Cancer Research UK (2003c) Tests you'll need. Updated 18 October 2001. Accessed from www.cancerresearchuk.org (18 November 2003).

Cancer Research UK (2003d) Your digestive system. Updated 19 May 2002. Accessed from www.cancerresearchuk.org (18 November 2003).

Cancer Research UK (2003e) Your mouth. Updated 19 October 2001. Accessed from www.cancerresearchuk.org (18 November 2003).

Corner J (1996) Non-pharmacological intervention for breathlessness in lung cancer. Palliative Medicine 10: 299-305.

Gerbrecht B-M (2003) Current Canadian experience with capecitabine: partnering with patients to optimize therapy. Cancer Nursing 26: 161-7.

Holmes S (1996) Chemotherapy: A guide for practice, 2nd edn. Dorking: Asset Books Ltd.

Holmes S (1997) The maintenance of health during radiotherapy: a nursing perspective. Journal of the Royal Society of Health 117: 393-9.

Kaye P (1994) A-Z Pocketbook of Symptom Control. Northampton: EPL Publications.

Markman M (1997) Basic Cancer Medicine. London: WB Saunders.

MIMS (2000) Handbook of Oncology. London: Medical Imprint/Janssen Cilag Ltd.

Moertel CG, Fleming TR, Macdonald JS (1990) Levamisole and fluorouracil for adjuvant therapy of resected colon carcinoma. New England Journal of Medicine 322: 352-8.

Morse J (1994) The phenomenology of comfort. Journal of Advanced Nursing 20: 189-95.

National Cancer Guidance Group (2004) Improving Outcomes in Colorectal Cancer: Updated manual. London: NICE.

NHS Executive (1997a) Improving Outcomes in Colorectal Cancer. London: HMSO.

NHS Executive (1997b) Improving Outcomes in Colorectal Cancer: The research evidence. London: HMSO.

Roberts DK, Thorne SE, Pearson C (1993) The experience of dyspnoea in late stage cancer: patients' and nurses' perspectives. Cancer Nursing 1: 310-20.

Roper N, Logan W, Tierney A (1996) The Elements of Nursing: A model for nursing based on a model of living, 4th edn. Edinburgh: Churchill Livingstone.

Rougier P, Van Cutsem E, Bajetta E (1998) Randomised trial of irinotecan versus fluorouracil by continuous infusion after fluorouracil failure in patients with metastatic colorectal cancer. The Lancet 352:1407-12.

Roy C (1984) Introduction To Nursing: An adaptation model. Englewood Cliffs, NJ: Prentice Hall.

Souhami R, Tobias J (1998) Cancer and its Management, 3rd edn. Oxford: Blackwell Science.

Weinberg RA (1998) One Renegade Cell. London: Weidenfeld & Nicolson.

Wolmark N, Rockette H, Fisher B (1993) The benefit of leucovorin-modulated fluorouracil as postoperative adjuvant therapy for primary colon cancer: results from National Surgical Adjuvant Breast and Bowel Project protocol C-03. Journal of Clinical Oncology 11: 1879-87.

Appendix

Antiemetic guidelines for chemotherapy-induced nausea and vomiting - an example

The combined use of antiemetic procedures and audit is becoming standard practice in many NHS trusts/local or national cancer networks in an attempt to measure and subsequently improve patient care (MIMS 2000, p. 67).

Management principles

Goals

- Ensure good first-time control, thereby reducing the risk of patient-induced anticipatory nausea and vomiting
- Establish patient susceptibility: factors that have shown to indicate poor antiemetic control include past experience of chemotherapy, age and gender
- Educate doctors and nurses involved in the prescribing and administration of cytotoxic drugs and their potential side effects
- Promote the appropriate use of antiemetic drugs; these should be given a minimum of 30 min before chemotherapy agents
- Encourage continuity of prescribing for optimal control

Key elements of antiemetic procedures

- Provide a sound definition of successful management
- Classify chemotherapy regimens:
  - low
  - low-moderate
  - high-moderate
  - higher risk treatments
- Provide a recognized list of potential factors, which could move patients from one antiemetic regimen, if they are perceived to be at a greater risk of developing nausea and vomiting (MIMS 2000, p. 67)

Chapter 7

Radiotherapy

Wendy Farrell

Radiotherapy is a specialized therapeutic option within the provision of cancer treatments. It has been stated that between 50 and 70% of all cancer patients will undergo radiotherapy as a treatment option during their cancer trajectory (Spence and Johnson 2001). It is therefore imperative that, as health-care professionals, we are knowledgeable about the provision of radiotherapy, the overall aim and intention of the treatment, and its potential adverse effects (Holmes 1996). This chapter aims to provide a synopsis of information about the use of radiotherapy in relation to bowel cancer and the consequences for the patient.

The underlying principles of radiotherapy and the consequential effects on normal and malignant cells are discussed. The process of receiving radiotherapy as a treatment is explored, highlighting current trends and recommendations for practice. Finally the potential effects that radiotherapy can have upon the patient, including the supportive care required by those patients undergoing treatment, are discussed.

Radiotherapy has various ways of helping the clinician treat the cancer patient. In effect, it has the ability to assist in the overall prognosis by promoting a curative response. Radiotherapy can provide an element of control and stability over the potential growth of disease, and finally it has the ability to assist in the palliation of symptoms of advanced cancers (Holmes 1996, Iwamoto 2001, Spence and Johnston 2001). Radiotherapy is not, however, always used as a 'stand-alone' treatment and is frequently used in conjunction with other forms of intervention, i.e. surgery and/or chemotherapy (Campbell and Farrell 1998), which can influence the effects of radiotherapy experienced by the patient.

What is radiotherapy?

Radiotherapy is the use of ionizing radiation. The underlying principles of its use as a viable treatment option are embedded within the application of radiation physics and radiobiology theories (Hilderley 1993).

Application of radiation physics

The underlying theory of radiation physics is based on the effects of radiation on the atomic structure. By using radiation, we depend on this form of energy interacting with atoms within the cells of our bodies, to produce particular biological effects. Such effects will then prove harmful and inhibit the normal functioning of the cells targeted. An atom has been described by Bomford et al. (1993) as a 'miniature solar system', as a result of its formation. Within the atom there is a nucleus, which contains protons and neutrons. Protons possess a positive charge, whereas neutrons possess no charge. Circulating around the nucleus are orbits (hence the solar system comparison), which carry electrons; there are equal numbers of electrons and protons present in the nucleus, the electrons carrying a negative charge. Electrostatic forces hold the atom together. It is this type of atom that is deemed stable.

All forms of radiation contain energy. When conducting a beam of radiation there is the potential to transfer this energy from the source to the material through which it is passing. Consequently, if a source of radiation is directed at tissues of the body, it is possible for the stability of the atom to be affected. This is achieved by the energy 'knocking out' an electron from an orbit; the subsequent energy released causes ionization of that atom. As a direct result of this, both the atom, which is now classed as being unstable, and the 'free' electron work together to bring about chemical changes within the cell; these changes are based on the interactions with DNA, which ultimately lead to the inability of the cell to function effectively and subsequently result in damage and death (Holmes 1996, Campbell and Farrell 1998).

There are two processes by which radiation can be delivered:

1. Electromagnetic radiation
2. Particulate radiation.

Electromagnetic radiation is the form used in radiotherapy, because of its properties. It has been found to have the shortest wavelength and to possess the greatest amount of energy, which will inevitably heighten the potential of interaction with the atomic structures. The two main forms of delivery are from either gamma rays or X-rays. Neither of these forms possesses a mass and consequently they have the ability to penetrate the tissues to a deeper level and release more radiation, which will have catastrophic effects on the ability of the atoms to remain stable and maintain normal functioning (Bomford et al. 1993, Hilderley 1993, Holmes 1996).

Application of radiobiology

The theory of radiobiology is based on the effects of radiation on the biological functioning of the cell after ionization. Within the body there are approximately 30 trillion (10^{12}) cells, which are dependent on a process of self-regulation and proliferation (Weinberg 1997). A normal cell reproduces when it is instructed to do so, whereas malignant cells disregard this process and replicate to their own agenda. This process of cell replication and proliferation is termed the 'cell cycle' (see Chapter 6). In conclusion, the use of therapies such as radiation and cytotoxic agents aims to disrupt this functioning process.

These principles of radiobiology are based on the ability of the cell to continue to replicate and proliferate. The greatest effects of radiation on cellular functioning occur within the stages of mitosis. The activity of the cells can be affected by the radiation in two ways: first there is a delay in the onset of the cycle, resulting in the potential for cell recovery, or complete inhibition, whereby the cells' actions cease and cells remain in a static state.

Although normal cells and malignant cells replicate in the same way, there are notable variations in the capabilities of their overall performance. These variations have been found to enhance the effectiveness of radiation on the cell cycle, especially when patients are receiving radiotherapy as a 'fractionated' course. This is when the patient receives a small daily dose of radiotherapy over a period of time, as opposed to receiving a large dose to a specific area once. These variations have been termed the '4 Rs of radiobiology' (Table 7.1) (Hilderley 1993, Holmes 1996, Campbell and Farrell 1998).

Repair is when normal cells have the ability to repair themselves; malignant cells, if they can be repaired, become re-oxygenated, thereby

Table 7.1 The 4 Rs of radiobiology

Repair
Redistribution
Repopulation
Re-oxygenation

increasing their vulnerability to radiation. Redistribution is when malignant cells are delayed in their activity through the cell cycle and subsequently are at the stage of mitosis when exposed to further radiation, which will heighten their sensitivity. Repopulation is the ability of normal cells to recover quickly before receiving another dose of radiation. It has been found that malignant cells can perform this only on rare occasions and as previously stated become re-oxygenated as a consequence. Being re-oxygenated is seen to be particularly hazardous for malignant cells. They are originally hypoxic in nature, which can be protective against radiation.

Radiotherapy is most effective on those tissues that are undifferentiated and well oxygenated, and those that actively replicate and proliferate. Areas within the body that are radiosensitive have been categorized by Holmes (1996) (Table 7.2). Consequently, identification of the gastrointestinal epithelium as a radiosensitive area promotes the use of radiotherapy within the treatment of colorectal cancers.

Table 7.2 Radiosensitive areas of the body

Hair follicles

Gastrointestinal epithelium

Genitourinary tract

Gonads

Bone marrow

Lymphoid tissue

From Holmes (1996, p. 32)

Current trends in practice in the provision of radiotherapy

In 1997, the NHS Executive published *Guidance on Commissioning Cancer Services, Improving Outcomes in Colorectal Cancer: The research evidence*. The document stated that radiotherapy played a significant part in the treatment of rectal cancer. Research suggested that radiotherapy undertaken preoperatively reduced the chance of local recurrence of disease (within the site of treatment) by up to 40%. The report also suggests that the overall 5-year survival rate could be increased up to 6% in those patients who underwent a curative resection. After the collation of these findings, several recommendations were made with regard to treatment by radiotherapy in the management of colorectal cancer within the UK.

These recommendations are summarized as follows:

1. All rectal cancer patients should receive radiotherapy if not contraindicated clinically.
2. Preoperative radiotherapy should be given unless the surgeon can ensure low local recurrence rates, i.e. ≤ 10%.
3. Patients who are considered high risk after surgery for potential recurrence should be considered for radiotherapy.
4. Patients receiving radiotherapy should have access to an experienced oncology nurse for support and information.

It can be proposed that rectal cancer often requires a combined modality approach to treatment, and this can be attributed to the limitation of the treatments for the disease; this in turn depends on the location and extent. Surgery rarely fails to reduce tumour bulk but cannot guarantee excision of microscopic disease, whereas radiotherapy is limited in its ability to reduce tumour size but has the potential to promote annihilation of microscopic disease. In effect, it could be said that the treatments complement each other. Glimelius (2001) reports that, in 20 randomized trials in which patients received surgery as a 'stand-alone' approach to the treatment of their disease, 20–28% of the patients experienced local recurrence. However, there may be situations when surgery is not possible; in these cases radiotherapy may provide an option to promote local control and cure through treatment with high-dose radiotherapy using endocavitary irradiation. This is because of the severe and acute toxicity that would be a consequence of the application of external beam radiotherapy (Gérard et al. 2003).

When considering the use of radiotherapy in the treatment of rectal cancer, it is important to recognize that there are options for its use, because radiotherapy can be given both pre- and postoperatively. Rectal cancers are often regarded as treatable by surgical resection; however, in some patients the extent of disease is beyond curative resection. Radiotherapy as an additional treatment has the potential to prevent disease recurrence (Glimelius 2001, Foroudi et al. 2003). Bujko and Nowacki (2002) propose that poor surgical technique, such as incomplete excision of a rectal tumour, could be viewed as the underlying cause of recurrence.

Treatment by radiotherapy can be categorized into two pathways: preoperatively and postoperatively. Glimelius (2001) stated that radiotherapy was not a suitable option for those patients who are deemed as low risk, i.e. their stage of disease was either T1 or T2 with no lymph node involvement, or those patients identified with metastatic disease on diagnosis. When debating the benefit of preoperative radiotherapy studies conclude that there was a 60–65% rate of reduction in localized disease recurrence, whereas the level achieved if given postoperatively could only realize between 20 and 40% (Glimelius 2001). The regimen for preoperative radiotherapy is widely discussed; traditionally this has been given as a long fractionated course (1.8 or 2.0 Gy given daily for 5 weeks).

Recent studies now promote the revision of such treatment regimens. The Swedish Rectal Cancer Trial (SRCT 1997) and the Dutch Total Mesorectal Excision (TME) Trial (Kapitejin et al. 2001) each advocate the use of a more intensive preoperative radiotherapy programme. Both trials indicate that treatment consisted of a higher dosage, shorter fractionated course (five fractions of 5 Gy), followed by prompt surgery (within 1 week of completion). This radical method of radiotherapy and timely surgery appeared to be fairly well tolerated by patients with minimal treatment toxicities.

The success of preoperative radiotherapy has contributed to the effects that radiotherapy has on the tumour cells, because the cells have a higher level of oxygenation before surgical intervention, thus heightening the sensitivity to radiotherapy. Radiotherapy has the ability to 'devitalize' those tumour cells thought to be responsible for metastatic spread after surgery (Peeters et al. 2003). The review on the impact of these trials concluded that this evidence, if used as a baseline, would prove to be effective, practical and prompt; as a consequence this approach is now widely accepted within Europe. It is necessary to note that only those tumours that are stage II or III rectal cancers would benefit from this type of regimen complemented by the original tumour location (Glynne-Jones and Sebag-Montefiore 2002).

A further treatment option is preoperative radiotherapy in combination with chemotherapy; however, patients experience a marked increase in the level of toxicity with this method. Irinotecan, a more recent addition to the cytotoxic range of drugs, is seen to contain radiosensitizing properties; together with preoperative radiotherapy it is reported as an effective regimen (Voelter et al. 2003) (see Chapter 6). However, irinotecan has a high risk of toxicity after treatment and one of the main adverse effects is diarrhoea, which may prove distressing and difficult for the patient to cope with. There is also the potential that the patient may experience an excessive amount of diarrhoea within the first 24 hours, and could potentially require hospital assessment or admission to control and monitor the effects.

The NHS Executive (1997) examined preoperative treatment regimens and concluded that there was no significant difference between giving a long or a short fractionated course of radiotherapy. The document also indicates that implementation of such a regimen would be governed by available resources. The preferred pathway indicates the shorter fractionated course.

Debate continues in the UK about the use of postoperative radiotherapy, which in contrast is the main treatment pathway within the USA. The main aim of postoperative radiotherapy is to assist the eradication of any residual microscopic disease after surgery, which could heighten the risk of local recurrence but may not prevent the development of distant metastases (Hampton 1993). Consensus was reached that postoperative radiotherapy given in conjunction with chemotherapy (usually 5-fluorouracil or 5FU based) could aid the abolition of any disseminated disease within the surgical site and surrounding area, thus preventing any microscopic spread of disease. Administration can be either by infusion or in bolus form. Oral agents such as the fluoropyrimidines, e.g. capecitabine, have the ability to mimic the actions of a continual 5FU infusion (Glynne-Jones and Sebag-Montefiore 2002, Souglakos et al. 2003) (see Chapter 6).

Hampton (1993) highlighted an alternative approach in which the patient receives radiotherapy both before and after surgery; this is often termed the 'sandwich technique'. It involves the patient receiving a low-dose course before surgery and a high-dose course after surgery, although this is not without complications. It is well documented that body tissues have a radiation tolerance level of the amount that can be sustained; giving radiation before surgery can be dose limiting for further postoperative treatment. There are other factors that can influence the effectiveness of such a regimen, such as the potential repopulation of malignant cells when treatment is delayed after surgery as a result of patient-related problems.

An intracavitary device can also deliver radiotherapy. Souhami and Tobias (1995) cite work by Papillion, in 1975, who treated a group of patients with rectal cancer using a radioactive intracavitary device (all tumours were mobile and within the lower part of the rectum). The results indicated that a 78% 5-year survival rate was achieved. Surgical intervention was not an option for these patients, based on their overall poor prognosis. Daniel (2001) also states that patients can receive an intraoperative fraction of radiotherapy during their surgical procedure to help the resolution of possible disseminated disease.

Finally, radiotherapy plays a major part in palliation. Symptoms associated with local recurrence of disease can be dramatic and debilitating, such as pain and bleeding. Radiotherapy can reduce the intensity of discomfort and offer patient relief from distressing problems; however, used in this way radiotherapy can pose a dilemma for the palliative care team. Should a patient have a relapse of the disease, an offer of secondary irradiation to the same site has not been well validated (Glimelius 2003). Radiotherapy is therefore given as a course to limit the level and amount of toxicity experienced by the patient.

Radiotherapy planning

As an optional treatment, radiotherapy is more powerful than an X-ray and requires meticulous preparation. There are a number of factors to be considered and each patient will have a specific treatment plan (Hilderley 1993). Patients are required to undergo rigorous investigations to provide a high level of information about their condition in preparation for the planning stage. These include a digital rectal examination, sigmoidoscopy, colonoscopy and barium enema. Scanning of the abdominal and pelvic regions is advantageous because this allows the extent of disease to be established, with the aim of identifying any distribution of metastatic disease. These investigations are vital because they can influence a patient's overall treatment. A clinical assessment will determine the current health and disease status, because these influence the patient's performance ability and ultimately the type of treatment offered (Dobbs et al. 1992).

There are several elements to be considered throughout the planning process. Based on the information obtained from the investigations, the tumour volume or the size of the area to be treated is identified. The target volume, for calculating the amount of treatment to be given, incorporates the tumour history and capability, i.e. the potential to spread; in effect a 'biological margin' is made around the tumour volume to assist with control of the disease (Dobbs et al. 1992). Another consideration in this procedure is patient position. This is a most imperative part of the planning process and therefore it is important to ensure that the position chosen is:

- comfortable for the patient
- technically appropriate
- documented effectively, to ensure that reproduction of the position can be exact.

During the planning process a machine called a simulator is used, which has the ability to mimic the actions of a radiotherapy machine and subsequently reproduce the treatment conditions before giving any treatment. To assist in subsequent positioning and alignment of the machine, patients are marked with either a specific waterproof marking pen or small 'tattoos', to ensure that they are not removed when washing.

At this stage the amount of radiation to be given has to be calculated. Dobbs et al. (1992) state that the effect of any given dose on the biological functioning of the cells is difficult to predict because of the lack of knowledge about cell density; these cells are situated in the centre and periphery of the target volume.

When planning radiotherapy for the rectal area, patients are placed in the prone position with a full bladder, which will displace the small bowel. Using a three-field technique the rectal region is treated; this ensures that the tumour receives radiation from all directions, which helps with treatment effectiveness. All three fields are treated daily (Dobbs et al. 1992).

Adverse effects of radiotherapy

As with any treatment, there is the potential for adverse effects on the individual, and radiotherapy is no exception. Radiotherapy cannot differentiate between normal and malignant cells, so the effects of radiotherapy are not confined to the treated area, which results in patients experiencing a level of toxicity (Campbell and Farrell 1998).

Much of the literature about the supportive care of patients undergoing radiotherapy states the importance of patient awareness of any potential adverse effects of the treatment and of the interventions that can be offered to alleviate their severity. It is imperative that all health-care professionals assess the individual needs of patients and their families, including comprehension of their current situation and the implications of treatment. Studies indicate that patients want information that is consistent and would prepare them for any eventuality that might occur during their treatment regimen. An ethical requirement is that patients need information if they are to give knowledgeable consent to treatment (Hilderley 1993, Hammick et al. 1998, Guren et al. 2003) (see Chapter 12).

The intensity of adverse effects depends on the treatment regimen; as previously discussed, those patients undergoing a short course of preoperative radiotherapy experience minimal problems and are able to withstand surgery. In fact, there is no evidence to suggest that a high toxicity level has been reported for the use of preoperative radiotherapy as a single agent. This differs considerably when combined with chemotherapy because patients can then experience significant problems (Crawshaw et al. 2003).

As a localized treatment, any side effects (Table 7.3) are usually confined to the treatment area but depend on a variety of factors, as noted by Holmes (1996).

Table 7.3 Factors influencing the occurrence of radiotherapy side effects

- The amount of tissue within the radiotherapy treatment field
- Tissues and organs that are present within the radiotherapy treatment field
- The radiosensitivity of the treatment area (those tissues and organs involved)
- Total dose of the radiation being given
- How the radiation is being given, i.e. single or fractionated course
- Energy of the radiation source
- Previous treatment, and concomitant surgery/chemotherapy
- Individual disease and health status

From Holmes (1996, p. 67)

It is important to acknowledge that any adverse effects reported are unique to each patient; some patients can have minimal disturbance and subsequently cope well with treatment, whereas others may present with a high level of toxicity and find sustaining treatment and its attributes extremely difficult (Holmes 1996). A further consideration is that these unpleasant reactions can be equally acute and chronic in their occurrence. This promotes the need for patients to be well supported throughout their treatment by individuals who are familiar and knowledgeable in the care/treatment regimen (NCGSG 2004).

Care of the patient undergoing radiotherapy

Skin irritation

One of the most common associated and discussed reactions of radiotherapy is attributed to damage inflicted on the basal layer of the epidermis by the radiation (Holmes 1996, Naylor and Mallett 2001). The body areas deemed most vulnerable are those that induce moisture and friction, i.e. the perineum, face and neck. These sites have a probability of contact between two skin layers, promoting friction and moisture. Skin reactions can manifest 2–3 weeks after the start of treatment and can take up to 1 month to resolve on completion of the treatment regimen. Studies estimate that up to 95% of patients will have a degree of skin reaction after treatment (De Conno et al. 1991 cited by Naylor and Mallett 2001, p. 231).

Education is seen as a vital part of patient preparation for any possible skin damage. Radiotherapy units offer relevant published and locally collated patient information on the topic.

The principles of an effective skin care routine can be summarized as follows:

- The use of perfumed soap and products on the area is not recommended.
- Avoid the area being exposed to direct sunlight.
- Wear loose cotton clothing around the area.
- Use only recommended creams for topical use to the treatment area, such as E45 cream, 1% hydrocortisone cream and prescribed creams if the level of reaction proves severe.
- Maintain and promote a good level of hygiene.

Naylor and Mallett (2001) identify four main stages of radiotherapy-induced reaction, which describe the status of skin integrity (Table 7.4). They also indicated that the occurrence and development of any reaction will progress during treatment. Frequent monitoring for skin integrity by the radiography team is important. The patient's treatment area or 'site' is inspected daily while being positioned for treatment. Some units use an assessment tool to gauge any problems and encourage a consistent approach in caring for such reactions. Any routine proposed will depend on the degree of skin trauma. Management of irradiated skin is much debated, with regard to the use of specific products including those no longer recommended. Some hospitals/units have their own treatment policy and these may differ from products usually indicated; also this could be influenced by consultant preference. However, Naylor and Mallett (2001) collated information about the use of treatments for skin reactions over the last decade and concluded that, for those reactions within stage 1 and 2, the use of moisturizing creams, e.g. E45 and also topical hydrocortisone (1%) cream/ointment, was often recommended. However, for the management of a stage 3 reaction, most of the clinical evidence indicated the use of a hydrocolloid sheet; this would prove successful if no infection were present at the site of the reaction. This literature review quite clearly stipulates what should not be used in the treatment of skin reactions: petroleum jelly, topical antibiotics when infection is not verified, topical steroids on stage 3 reactions and gentian violet – a traditional method of treating reactions.

Table 7.4 Stages of skin reactions to the use of radiotherapy

Stage	Presentation
1	Erythema: warmth, redness, local irritation
2	Dry desquamation: skin becomes dry, irritated, cracking and flaking
3	Moist desquamation: blistering, oedema, exudate, painful, infected
4	Necrosis: death of the tissue within the area

From Naylor and Mallett (2001, p. 231).

Diarrhoea

This is extremely common for patients treated with radiotherapy to the pelvic or abdominal fields; it is largely attributed to the effect on and damage to the intestinal mucosal layer. The occurrence of this problem progresses throughout the duration of treatment, subsequently increasing in severity. Patients need advice on their dietary and fluid intake, including the importance of recording and reporting the frequency of bowel actions. Consumption of a low-residue diet can assist the patient in tolerance of this alteration in bowel activity (see Chapter 11). The use of anti-spasmodic medication may also help in the regulation of bowel movement. Health professionals working in either primary or secondary care need to monitor these patients, to ensure that they retain adequate hydration and that any weight loss caused by the increased bowel actions and dietary changes is kept to a minimum. The importance of maintaining skin integrity in these circumstances is paramount because this can compound the severity of the existing skin damage. The patient with diarrhoea and a stoma needs specific advice and surveillance as a result of the impact on the stoma site and management (see Chapter 9).

Nausea and vomiting

The potential for patients to experience nausea and vomiting during their treatment regimen is subjective. First, this can depend on the area or treatment field. The likelihood of nausea and vomiting is more apparent when patients are undergoing radiotherapy to a large abdominal area. Patient assessment encourages compliance on the use of regular antiemetic drugs, which may be prescribed before treatment to combat post-treatment nausea and vomiting.

Fatigue

This is a common symptom associated with any type of radiotherapy, irrespective of field. It is not fully understood why patients experience such a high level of fatigue. The nature of fatigue is progressive throughout the duration of treatment and for 1–2 months after completion. (Guren et al. 2003). Associated effects of the treatment regimen can increase the occurrence of fatigue. It is important for patients and their families to understand fully and appreciate how debilitating the level of fatigue is and the implications for their daily routine.

Murphy (2001) examined the issue of radiotherapy for rectal tumours and concluded that there are several potential problems associated with the treatment. Some of these have already been discussed; others that can occur include proctitis, cystitis, sexual dysfunction and bone marrow suppression. However, not all patients are affected with every acknowledged side effect; similarly those unpleasant reactions vary in their level of intensity between patients. This reinforces the significance of a team approach to deliver individualized patient care throughout the treatment programme and ongoing surveillance.

Summary

Radiotherapy is seen as an integral part in the treatment of bowel cancer, especially rectal cancer. It is multifaceted and can be used in many ways and at various times throughout the patient's cancer trajectory. As an optional treatment it is complex as a result of the potential effect of radiation at a cellular level. In effect, preparation for treatment requires exact planning and delivery to ensure and promote patient well-being. Patient compliance depends on individual comprehension and readiness to undertake a treatment that will undoubtedly affect them adversely.

Overall conclusion

The use of radiotherapy has been debated through the instigation and use of clinical trials, and subsequently treatment regimens are now changing to promote treatment delivery, which is evidence-based. Radiotherapy is currently viewed as a desirable asset, which can be implemented in many ways to promote its overall treatment success for patients and consequent effects on cancer survival. Several trials are examining the combination of different treatment styles and their effectiveness on local control and potential cure. In spite of scientific advances in treatment provision, it is inevitable that patients will be at risk from unpleasant side effects. Health professionals are required by their professional organization to maintain their knowledge about current practice, policies and procedures relating to all aspects of radiotherapy administration, empowering patients and their families to be conversant and supported throughout their treatment journey (Nursing and Midwifery Council or NMC 2002).

Summary of key points

- Integral part of treating cancer: radiotherapy is one of the main forms of treatment within cancer care due to its potential effects upon cancer.
- Used in many ways: radiotherapy has the ability to be delivered in a variety of means, i.e. internally and externally, and by single fractions, or as short or long fractionated courses dependent on the desired effect of treatment and the potential adverse effects on the patient.
- Complex in its effects upon the body: this relates to how the radiotherapy affects the functioning of the cells by the four Rs.
- Requires precision planning and delivery: there is a definitive need to ensure that the patient is prepared and that the area to be treated is ready so that adverse effects can be minimized and organs and other vulnerable areas of the body protected; it also ensures that the patient receives the correct dose of radiation.

- Variety of potential adverse effects: depending on the type of radiotherapy given, the length of the course and the area being treated will influence the experience of adverse effects.

References

Bomford CK, Kunkler IH, Sherriff SB (1993) Walter and Miller's Textbook of Radiotherapy. Radiation Physics, Therapy and Oncology, 5th edn. London: Churchill Livingstone.

Bujko K, Nowacki MP (2002) Emerging standards of radiotherapy combined with radical rectal cancer surgery. Cancer Treatment Reviews 28: 101–13.

Campbell T, Farrell W (1998) Palliative radiotherapy for advanced cancer symptoms. International Journal of Palliative Nursing 4: 292–9.

Crawshaw A, Hennigan T, Smedley FH et al. (2003) Peri-operative radiotherapy for rectal cancer: the case for a selective pre-operative approach – the third way. Colorectal Disease 5: 367–72.

Daniel BT (2001) Gastrointestinal cancers. In: Otto SE (ed.), Oncology Nursing, 4th edn. St Louis: Mosby, Chapter 9.

De Conno F, Ventafridda V, Saita L (1991) Skin problems in advanced and terminal cancer patients. Journal of Pain and Symptom Management 6: 247–56

Dobbs J, Barrett A, Ash D (1992) Practical Radiotherapy Planning, 2nd edn. London: Edward Arnold.

Foroudi F, Tyldesley S, Barbera L et al. (2003) An evidence-based estimate of the appropriate radiotherapy utilization rate for colorectal cancer. International Journal of Radiation Oncology, Biology and Physics 56: 1295–307.

Gérard JP, Romestaing P, Baulieux J et al. (2003) Local curative treatment of rectal cancer by radiotherapy alone. Colorectal Disease 5: 442–4.

Glimelius B (2001) Pre- or postoperative radiotherapy in rectal cancer – more to learn? Radiotherapy and Oncology 61: 1–5.

Glimelius B (2003) Recurrent rectal cancer. The pre-irradiated primary tumour: can more radiotherapy be given? Colorectal Disease 5: 501–3.

Glynne-Jones R, Sebag-Montefiore D (2002) Rectal cancer: Editorial. Rectal cancer: what can we learn from the Dutch TME Study? How will this study impact on current practice in the UK? Clinical Oncology 14: 170–3.

Guren MG, Dueland S, Skovlund E et al. (2003) Quality of life during radiotherapy for rectal cancer. European Journal of Cancer 39: 587–94.

Hammick M, Tutt A, Tait DM (1998) Knowledge and perception regarding radiotherapy and radiation in patients receiving radiotherapy: a qualitative study. European Journal of Cancer Care 7: 103–12.

Hampton B (1993) Gastrointestinal cancer: colon, rectum, and anus. In: Groenwald SL, Hansen Frogge M et al. (eds), Cancer Nursing Principles and Practice, 3rd edn. Boston: Jones & Bartlett, Chapter 42.

Hilderley LJ (1993) Radiotherapy. In: Groenwald SL, Hansen Frogge M et al. (eds), Cancer Nursing Principles and Practice, 3rd edn. Boston: Jones & Bartlett, Chapter 13.

Holmes S (1996) Radiotherapy: A guide for practice. Surrey: Asset Books.

Iwamoto R (2001) Radiation Therapy. In: Otto SE (ed.), Oncology Nursing, 4th edn. St Louis: Mosby, Chapter 22.

Kapitejin E, Marijnen CAM, Nagtegaal IM et al. for the Dutch ColoRectal Cancer Group and other cooperative investigators (2001) Preoperative radiotherapy in combination with total mesorectal excision improves local control in respectable rectal cancer. Report for a multicenter randomised trial. New England Journal of Medicine 345: 638–46.

Murphy ME (2001) Colorectal cancers. In: Otto SE (ed.), Oncology Nursing, 4th edn. St Louis: Mosby, Chapter 8.

National Cancer Guidance Steering Group (2004) Improving Outcomes in Colorectal Cancer: Updated manual. London: NICE.

Naylor W, Mallett J (2001) Management of acute radiotherapy induced skin reactions: a literature review. European Journal of Oncology Nursing 5: 221-33.

NHS Executive (1997) Guidance on Commissioning Cancer Services. Improving Outcomes in Colorectal Cancer. The research evidence. London: Department of Health.

Nursing and Midwifery Council (2002) Code of Professional Conduct. London: NMC.

Papillion J (1975) Intracavity irradiation of early rectal cancer for cure. Cancer 36: 696-701.

Peeters KCMJ, Kapiteijn E, Van de Velde CJH (2003) Managing rectal cancer: the Dutch experience. Colorectal Disease 5: 423-6.

Souglakos J, Androulakis N, Mavroudis D et al. (2003) Multicentre dose-finding study of concurrent capecitabine and radiotherapy as adjuvant treatment for operable rectal cancer. International Journal of Radiation Oncology, Biology and Physics 56: 1284-7.

Souhami R, Tobias J (1995) Cancer and its Management, 2nd edn. Avon: Blackwell Science.

Spence RAJ, Johnston PG (eds) (2001) Oncology. Oxford: Oxford University Press.

Swedish Rectal Cancer Trial (SRCT) (1997) Improved survival with perioperative radiotherapy in resectable rectal cancer. New England Journal of Medicine 336: 980-7.

Voelter V, Stupp R, Matter M et al. (2003) Preoperative hyperfractionated accelerated radiotherapy (HART) and concomitant CPT-11 in locally advanced rectal carcinoma: A phase I study. International Journal of Radiation Oncology, Biology and Physics 56: 1288-94.

Weinberg RA (1997) How cancer arises. In: Freeman WH (ed.), What you Need to Know About Cancer. New York: Scientific American.

Part 3

Management and care of patients with bowel cancer

Chapter 8

Psychosocial aspects of care

Barbara Borwell

Case study

I came across Jean in the hospital coffee bar. Our association began when fund raising for a local cancer charity. An emotional Jean explained that Peter was in hospital having been diagnosed with bowel cancer and needing a colostomy. The operation was tomorrow and she was sitting there, not knowing what to say, who to tell or what to do, hoping to put on a 'brave face', not wishing to cause Peter any additional anxiety. 'All these years we've been fund-raising its different when it happens to you, this is the side you don't know or hear about. It's not fair.'

This chapter explores the potential impact of colorectal cancer (CRC) during the many phases in the development of the disease. A diagnosis of cancer is associated with substantial patient psychological morbidity. Between 10 and 20% will develop a recognized psychiatric condition (Barraclough 1997). The many associated psychosocial problems are recognized in the Department of Health's document on the commissioning of cancer services (Expert Advisory Group on Cancer 1995) which describes a network of services from primary care through hospital cancer units to cancer centres. *The NHS Cancer Plan* also acknowledges that the cancer journey has a devastating effect on patients and carers, highlighting the patient experience as a priority and central to care (DoH 2000).

Recommendations include the need for psychosocial support for individuals, although the specificity about what these psychosocial needs are and how support should be provided is less clear.

Throughout the life cycle people face expected challenges such as marriage and retirement; others can be unexpected life crises such as sudden death or other personal tragedy. Families may already be coping with these unexpected events when they have to face the additional strain caused by receiving bad news. A diagnosis of colorectal cancer in one family member changes the emotional stability, responsibilities, financial status and social interactions of the spouse and partner as well as the remainder of the family. The quality of the relationship before diagnosis can be a determinant of the distress felt by the carer (Frude 1991). Any previous history of major life crises such as bereavement, mental illness or major physical illness, and the ability of the family unit to cope, are indicators of how they will cope with additional stress. Several studies indicate that the extended family of friends, community, spiritual and employment associates, and local resources contribute to the rehabilitation process (Krishnasamy 1996, McGreachy 2001).

Cancer in the twenty-first century is still seen by many patients as a 'death sentence' linked with stigma and intractable pain, having a profound psychological effect on the functioning ability of both the patient and the family. The initial reaction produces a psychological crisis, which may cause fear, anxiety, disbelief, anger and depression, leading to anguish and vulnerability. As patients search for a meaning and try to take 'control' of the situation, a wide range of responses is encountered. Health professional interventions can focus on physical care, but of paramount significance is an understanding of those factors that help to maintain the quality of life.

Psychosocial care is concerned with the psychological and emotional well-being of the patient, the family and carers, who live and work in a multicultural society. Considerations include issues of self-esteem, insight into and adaptation to the disease and its consequences, communication, social functioning and relationships (National Council for Hospices and Specialist Palliative Care Units 2002). The giving of information, Cobbs (1976) noted, should relate to maintaining respected status and personal value, 'belonging to a network of communication and obligation'.

Increased awareness of psychosocial problems has led to numerous therapeutic approaches to interventions for patients and their families, from informal and formal listening skills through to complementary therapies, such as art and aromatherapy (see Chapter 13) provided by friends, trained volunteers or professionals. The value of counselling and support by specialist nurses working as part of a multidisciplinary team is recognized in the management and routine care of cancer patients (NHS Executive 1997). With the holistic approach, all health professionals need to have interpersonal competence, combining cognitive, behavioural *and* communication skills. The nurse–patient relationship is especially important in cancer care (NHS Executive 1997), and may be a factor in cancer survival (Fallowfield 1995, Fawzy et al. 1995), although stress in the nursing staff can be doubly harmful (Kasch 1986, cited in Roberts and Snowball 1999).

Holistic care (Figure 8.1) acknowledges the physical, social, emotional and spiritual dimensions that are appropriate and central to the individual, with a growing recognition of associated distress. This jigsaw reminds us how all the pieces should fit to achieve optimum care.

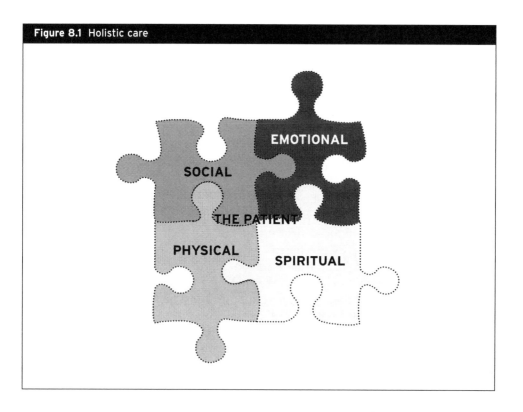

Figure 8.1 Holistic care

Social aspects of care

Changes in a patient's role in life, such as employment and relationships, are inevitable. Considerations include the capacity to fulfil and function in usual roles; in addition new roles will evolve, while existing relationships operate in a modified way (Shell and Kirsch 2001). The impact of financial and other concerns may cause stressors, which link to the many inevitable losses and changes taking place in a comparatively short period; these are compounded by immediate and future practical concerns such as the inability to continue with employment, hospital transportation costs, personal insurance or dietary needs (see Chapter 14).

Who to tell or should I tell?

Timing of information giving should be patient led, to enable acknowledgement of the situation. Most families operate as an interactive group, by sharing information, which enables a patient's supportive network time to nurture openness and the freedom to sustain each other. What cannot be overlooked are the stressors placed on the family. Cancer can be seen as a social phenomenon, a disease irrespective of age or gender generally associated with pain, mutilation and death. Personal reactions of those significant to the patient are usually determined by feelings about the person and disease, and beliefs and individual attitudes. Families may have negative feelings towards cancer and its management, but display an optimistic attitude when with the patient. This conflicting behaviour and false reassurances are not conducive to well-being. Junior members of the family unit should not be excluded; their level of involvement is determined by individual circumstances (Cancerlink 1994, cited in Borwell 1996, p. 52).

Social processes surrounding the health and well-being of cancer patients can be influenced in many ways by helping to promote healthy patterns of behaviour, strengthening their identity while searching for a meaning in life. It cannot be assumed that the patient will know *or* appreciate the various social support symptoms that are to hand. Attempts to identify and provide appropriate support must be founded on knowledge-based assessments which sustain the integrity of individual networks, consideration being given to those best equipped to meet particular needs (Norbeck 1981).

Emotional aspects of care

The psychological impact of cancer can be enormous. Bad news can dislocate daily activities and introduce doubt, all of which can threaten patients' physical and psychological well-being. According to Buckman (1992, p. 11) the 'badness' of bad news and its influence depend on what the patient already knows or suspects about the future. It is necessary to recognize high levels of psychological stress in the patient (and in the family/friends) between investigation and diagnosis, and between diagnosis and treatment (Shontz 1975). The incidence of psychological morbidity is estimated to be between 25 and 50%; related factors include anxiety, depression and fears associated with death, uncertainty, mutilation and altered self-concept (Hopwood and Stephens 2000). Psychological distress initially experienced by cancer victims and their close families is often compared with the 'grieving process' and mourning of the many consequential losses. Validation of the feelings and sadness that may be experienced, including 'the normality' attached to such reactions, can have a beneficial effect on the quality of life. This major life crisis confronts a patient with two significant threats. The impact of the disease and treatment can be viewed as a violation of body intactness, where a 'new body image' may need to be incorporated into an individual's 'self perception' (Price 1998; see also Chapter 9).

The psychosocial response to changes associated with cancer and mutilating surgery is therefore complex and highly individual, described by Hopson (1981) as transitions – a life event creating discontinuity, after which they will never be the same again. This discontinuity has two aspects:

1. The general consensus (sociocultural)
2. The person's own perception.

A summary of Hopson's (1981) description of the general and personal aspects of the situation, and his identification of seven transitions within it before final acceptance, are as follows:

1. Immobilization: where patients are overwhelmed, shocked and unable to make plans, from which they gradually recover.

2. Minimization: the tendency to trivialize and deny the transition and its consequences. Denial, although usually temporary, is one of the most radical adaptive response mechanisms against reality in serious or terminal illness: 'this can't be true'. Every patient at some time will experience denial, more so at the start of a serious illness than towards the end of life (Buckman 1992). As this dissipates, high energy levels can often be demonstrated to maintain the mechanism of denial. This is not suppression but a means of coping. At this time patients may talk of their illness as a minor ailment, dismissing the apparent seriousness of the condition, but at the same time submitting themselves to the most radical of treatments.

3. Depression: as the individual becomes more fully aware of the extent of change and powerlessness. When denial can no longer be maintained, it is replaced by feelings of anger, envy, rage and resentment. Family and professionals become targets of disarticulation, as a result of an utter sense of helplessness and the acceptance of helplessness by others, which forms the basis for rage. This hostile behaviour can be fed by professionals' personal reactions to rage, which include employing avoidance tactics to shun confrontation. Depression is used to describe a more *chronic* state of mood and is known to be provoked by the threat of serious illness, when it becomes more than an adjustment disorder (Buckman 1992). Most people would expect depression to be an expectation following a cancer diagnosis. Advances in the treatment of cancer mean that patients are living longer with their illness, with potentially complex needs. The manifestation of the clinical disorder of depression is more than one would reasonably expect, emphasizing the importance of prompt diagnosis and treatment (Buckman 1992, Sheldon 1997).

4. 'Letting go': the individual slowly begins to accept the future reality, sometimes with optimism.

5. Testing: signals more energy as the individual begins to try out new coping strategies. This can lead to frustration when ideas and perceptions of how things should be do not progress as hoped.

6. A search for meaning looks at the reasons for life being different and change at this stage is accepted at the cognitive level. Underlying psychological dynamics may be associated with guilt; frequently by unsuccessful resolution of the previous phases an individual can delay the inevitable happening. Only when guilt is sensitively pursued can these irrational fears be alleviated.

7. Internalization occurs when the previous stage of searching has developed into behavioural change, leading to resolution and acceptance. The reality of illness can no longer be denied, once anger dissolves and the delusion of postponement ceases; this is substituted with a sense of great loss, anxiety and depression at changeable levels.

Holmes and Rahe (1967) assess readjustment in terms of the level of stress generated. The transition is usually surgery. In every case the patient must review his or her personal situation and accept lasting change, doing this quickly with no time to adjust psychically. This is difficult if as yet there is no feeling of illness. There may be extreme mood swings (similar to grieving) and the patient will need help to:

- review and change his or her personal constructs
- accept these changes
- gain a perception of the timescale for adjustment e.g. elective vs. emergency surgery (Parkes 1993).

Consequently, the type of intervention, such as stoma versus no stoma, will incur changes to an individual's body, with potential psychological difficulties for both the patient and the partner.

Cancer is commonly viewed as a stigmatizing condition; a stoma can emphasize this (Macdonald and Anderson 1984). Life satisfaction can be greatly affected by the disease and in some instances intervention can be anticipated with relief, a resolution to any discomfort and embarrassment often caused by advanced symptoms of disease. Equally, people who feel well and mainly symptom free before diagnosis can experience profound shock and panic when told they have cancer. Proposed interventions are not a primary concern until the reality of mutilating surgery and caring for a stoma is evident. Changes imposed by a 'life event' will not automatically progress in such a linear way. For most people the path can be equated to a pendulum, moving backwards and forwards until internalization is attained. These processes can mirror the grieving process.

Spirituality

The concept of spirituality and the provision of spiritual care are generally fraught with anxiety and difficulties for health-care staff. Within nursing the spiritual dimension of care is frequently expressed, consensus of opinion suggesting that nurses should discuss the spiritual needs of their patients – not unlike sexual needs, a frequently neglected aspect of care. Given the cultural and religious notion and diversity of spirituality, some faith traditions may be offended by the term 'spirituality' in health care. Others may take on a more humanistic, existential meaning (McSherry and Ross 2002, p. 481).

Understanding spirituality

The idea of patients having spiritual needs makes many nurses nervous. They need to recognize that the spiritual dimension is an important part of emotional strength. Spiritual does not necessarily mean 'religious' and this area does not have to be the province only of clergy. Think of it as a right to hold certain attitudes and to value certain things and/or practices. A feeling of confidence, safety and the opportunity for individual practice is necessary to the patient's well-being and contributes to healing (McSherry and Ross 2002).

Spirituality encompasses the whole range of life experiences, embracing culture, environment, work, family and social life, everything that reflects the uniqueness of each individual and the ability to react to life events and circumstances. Additional characteristics include the influence by and existence of family members, relationships and social backgrounds. Their attitudes, fears, hopes, strengths, weaknesses and coping abilities uniquely affect the individual, and his or her perception and experience. Addressing the spiritual aspects of care means offering care that is unique to individual needs. As previously stated individual variations are portrayed in many ways, either openly or at times not expressed but recognised intuitively. Providing opportunities for unconditional space in a safe environment, acknowledging uniqueness and conveying acceptance of an individual's beliefs and values are the progressive way to establish a patient's spiritual needs.

Cultural and religious aspects of spiritual care

Without an appreciation of the diversity and provision of support, nurses may undermine the social relationship at a time when most patients need to harness all their potential resources to help them cope with the disease

(Krishnasamy 1996). The potential impact of individual and family influences associated with culture, ethnic and religious background should be recognized by the multidisciplinary team. Within Europe the UK is regarded as one of the most ethnically distinct countries (Le Var 1998). There must be no discrimination, even unconscious, against religious observance and attitudes. Care should be taken not to assume that, or behave as though, any religion of the care team is superior to that of the patient. The team must have sensitive training and support on this point.

Religious beliefs and practices for many people are an important aspect of their spiritual care.

Patient assessment forms acknowledge religion but the matter of denomination is not pursued, and yet religious practices and beliefs may play an important part in daily life. Conversely, the significance of the religious denomination may only denote membership of a local community. Health-care workers should be conversant with and have insight into other religious practices, attitudes and denominations, particularly within in the local population served. However, parity in certain faiths cannot be resolute (Henley and Schott 1999).

Traditions, beliefs and attitudes of each cultural group can influence an individual's response to illness and nursing intervention for a condition such as bowel cancer. Orthodox Sikhs, for example, would not openly discuss with their spouse problems relating to bowels or genitourinary systems. Body waste is seen as polluting; the left hand is reserved for 'unclean tasks' and the right hand used for 'clean tasks' such as greeting and eating. Transcultural interventions by professionals should be sensitive and representative of the diverse cultural needs of patients and those significant in the family or society group. Cultural needs are determined as: equality of access to treatment and care; respect for cultural beliefs and practices, including: dietary, personal care, religious and daily routines; communication; and cultural safety needs (Narayanasamy 2003, p. 185).

Giving spiritual care

Multiprofessional team working enables any member to contribute and support a patient's spiritual needs. The nature of nursing, the bonding relationship and closeness developed between nurse and patient suggest that nurses are more likely to offer spiritual care while addressing other essential needs. The family contribution and support should also be observed and respected. Attending to the spiritual needs should start at the individual's place within the spiritual journey, addressing often difficult questions about cancer, the future, death and dying. It is about being empathic, facilitating permission to express what is happening in 'their world'.

Many cancer patients will seek connections while trying desperately to make sense of all that is happening, convincing themselves that God is cruel, or that they are sinners unable to understand that some things happen without reason. Searching for a meaning in the light of illness is a search of differing expressions, often with no results. Many individuals struggle to comprehend and conceptualize meaning and, as studies suggest, this is significant to the cancer experience (Taylor 1993). Any member of the care team (even the most junior) and the family may minister in this way. Empathy is the key, and often invites the voicing of doubts (and beliefs). This is an important *listening* area, even though no answers may be offered by the carers. It can help the patient to sort out his or her own thoughts. The interdenominational services of the hospital chaplain team are a source of support for both the patient and the staff. The importance of spiritual care has to be recognized for the potential whole healing force of body, mind and spirit. Understanding the dimensions of spirituality is fundamental if care plans are to reflect patient needs (Stoter 2002).

Sexuality

Sexuality spans all the elements of holistic care. The major core of human values lies in the philosophy of religion, sexuality and ethics. Cultural norms prescribe what behaviour is acceptable combined with rules (implicit and explicit) governing its expression. Serious illness and hospitalization can prompt a patient to reconsider life. Sexual behaviour can be viewed as an outcome of both society and culture (Woods and Lamb 1981), in addition to its biological origin. Sexuality may be affected in any surgery, but especially as close to home as the colorectal area. Hence, this is a source of great anxiety to patients and their families. In a multicultural society, attitudes, practices and custom on what may be voiced vary enormously.

In addition feelings about embarrassment-inducing changes in body image can adversely affect a patient's sexuality. There are problems of self-esteem because the patient's physical appearance does not conform to what is accepted and admired. The modern cult of visual perfection is responsible for much of this stress. Emphasis placed on the physical appearance will finally affect the self-perception of body image changes. This apparent physical problem suddenly transforms into a psychological dilemma, threatening relationships and friendship. Any hint of abnormality or disfigurement is shameful and inhibiting, although in some relationships there can be an increase in emotional stability. These effects can continue throughout the course of the disease and its treatment. Little thought is paid to the psychological repercussions of the terminology associated with cancer. Phrases such as malignancy and disease can affect the behaviour of patients and significant others. Health professionals must carefully define and clarify what is cancer and identify an individual's perception of how this might affect him or her and the family.

There are many ways in which a partner's illness can lead to a decrease or cessation of sexual contact. Disfigurement in any form and treatment side effects such as discomfort or fatigue may delay the resumption of sexual activity or closeness. Conversely, other couples find that a cancer diagnosis strengthens relationships and intimacy. To overcome fears of rejection, the importance of discussion about these potential side effects with patients and significant others within the relationship is paramount. Care must also be given to this aspect where there is no apparent partner. Nor should personal judgements be made about a patient's sexual orientation or that all couples are heterosexual. Homosexuals in or out of a relationship will experience similar concerns about the effects of cancer on sexual function as a heterosexual couple, requiring counselling and support. It is not within the professionals' remit to concentrate on a patient's sexual preference but to address sexual health issues related to colorectal cancer and its treatment.

Possible effects of bowel cancer on sexual health

Male

The possibility of sperm banking is mentioned. Erectile dysfunction may occur in men undergoing radical pelvic surgery such as abdominal excision of resection, or pelvic exenteration as a result of nerve or vascular damage (see Chapter 5). Bowel cancer is usually associated with the older person; however, occasionally a younger male can be diagnosed. Spermatogenesis may be affected by high-dose radiotherapy with arbitrary recovery (see Chapter 7).

Female

Multiple problems are associated with pelvic irradiation, including vaginal stenosis, dyspareunia, vaginal vault necrosis, decreased lubrication, fistulae and vaginal shortening. Surgical intervention such as abdominal excision of resection may result in alteration of pelvic anatomy, causing coital difficulties such as with penetration, scarring and discomfort (see Chapter 5). Treatment by some chemotherapeutic agents can increase the vulnerability to vaginal infections with susceptibility to odour and reduction in self-esteem (see Chapter 6).

Assumptions must not be made that the existence of a medical problem eradicates sexual needs. Initial assessment should establish any sexual dysfunctional problems relating to other conditions such as diabetes or previous surgery unrelated to the cancer, including the degree of sexual satisfaction currently experienced. Other causes related to disturbance of sexual function could be biological, physiological or neurological in nature, affecting sexual response and the concept of body image. Sexuality is inextricably linked to quality of life for both sexes.

Help in sexual matters

The assessment of sexuality for patients undergoing disfiguring cancer treatments, whether temporary or permanent, is an integrated part of care. As with spirituality, many nursing carers lack confidence in this area because they lack training in comfortable conversation with patients on sexuality (Williams 1986, Borwell 1997a, 1997b). A useful guide for busy practitioners, recognized by the Royal College of Nursing (RCN 2000), is an adaptation of the PLISSIT model (Anon 1976, Borwell 1997b). The important contribution by professionals is recognized in relation to their specific role and level of proficiency.

PLISSIT is an acronym, which when translated means:

Permission
Limited information
Specific suggestions
Intensive therapy.

Permission

This allows the topic of sexuality to be addressed through open questioning, enabling the patient or couple to voice any concerns about cancer affecting their relationship. This is also an opportunity for nurses to discuss any side effects of cancer therapies with regard to sexual function.

Limited information

This is the educational element where specific information can be given on the implications of treatment, with appropriate literature as additional support or other resources.

Specific suggestions

Previously identified issues can require more detailed information or advice, such as the use of a vaginal lubricant for dyspareunia or discussion of other forms of sensual love making. At this level, the nurse may feel less competent to address the issues raised, but able to refer to others.

Intensive therapy

Those issues have been identified that require the specific expertise of a psychosexual counsellor and referral is offered.

Physical problems associated with CRC vary depending on the presentation phase of the disease. Some patients may be asymptomatic with diagnosis prompted by attendance at a colorectal screening programme (see Chapter 2); others can present with changes affecting their usual pattern of elimination (see Chapter 5) before medical advice is sought. Depending on the severity of symptoms and their impact on daily life, e.g. fatigue, individuals will have either extreme or little concern in relation to the probable seriousness of their condition. The experience of distressing symptoms can prompt individuals either to seek advice or conversely to bury their heads in the sand in denial, even though highly anxious about the outcome. Some will have experienced little or no symptoms and 'feel well'. A cancer diagnosis and the implications of aggressive treatment can be overwhelming. Lack of or nominal information between investigations and diagnosis can induce high levels of anxiety, suggesting that the time from investigation to diagnosis should be kept to a minimum (Northouse 1989).

Patient information needs

The Department of Health has officially acknowledged that cancer patients have health needs, which include psychosocial as well as disease and treatment needs. National and locally agreed waiting-time targets, including pre-planned and pre-booked appointments for every patient diagnosed with cancer, have now been established (see earlier). Some will have sought professional advice while awaiting confirmation of the diagnosis. Others may find the territory alarming, declining contact or information.

The full, free and sensitive flow of information to cancer patients is an essential part of care; it is NHS policy that patients are treated as equal citizens throughout the cancer journey (DoH 2000, National Cancer Guidance Steering Group or NCGSG 2004).

The task of imparting timely information, whether good or bad, is now accepted by professionals as one of their responsibilities. The information process should include recognition of a patient's right to know the diagnosis, treatment options and outcomes, and how the cancer might affect other aspects of life, thus promoting patient autonomy (see Chapter 12). The establishment of care partnerships with patients enables them to determine the level of involvement in relation to decision-making and care.

A cancer diagnosis produces anxiety, which impairs the assimilation and retention of information. Reaction to 'bad news' is difficult to predict, indicating that information attainment pertaining to diagnosis and treatment options is variable. As a result of the anxiety factor, and varying levels of education, however, patients and families may require help to understand their situation and accept it (Mills and Sullivan 1999). Nursing involvement in providing and coordinating multidisciplinary communication and a contribution to the 'care package' is paramount to well-being. Professionals are usually governed by a code of conduct that establishes the role that morality plays in their specialist professions (see Chapter 12). CRC often affects those patients with special needs and yet these are often poorly met, both in hospital and in primary care. Hart (1998) explored the personal experiences of people with learning disabilities and highlighted a number of concerns, including hospital phobia, communication difficulties and unsatisfactory care. Carers, whether professional or family, may wish to be involved in the consultation, because they undoubtedly will have concerns, or feel a sense of responsibility. It is important to establish that the patient is in agreement with this. Sometimes the presence of a carer will increase patient confidence, especially when important information has to be communicated. Consensus among most cancer patients and informal carers indicates that patients want substantial information, acknowledging that specific needs will vary (Fallowfield et al. 1994).

Nursing assessment should not discriminate between the essential needs of a multicultural, often older, patient group. In their study Graydon et al. (1997, p. 60) used the breast cancer version of the Toronto Informational Needs Questionnaire to measure the information needs about the experience of having cancer. An adapted version for bowel cancer is outlined in Table 8.1. Profiling will also help to establish appropriate information and support needs perceived as important to individuals and their families, identifying those not wishing to know the truth about their condition.

Table 8.1 Informational needs assessment tool (an example)

Please read the following statements and circle the number which best describes how important it is for you to be given this information:

1 = not important   2 = slightly important   3 = moderately important   4 = very important
5 = extremely important

It is important for me to know	Not important				Very important
How I will feel during/after investigations	1	2	3	4	5
How to prepare for my treatment	1	2	3	4	5
Who I should contact if I have any concerns during treatment	1	2	3	4	5
How bowel cancer and the treatment affects my body	1	2	3	4	5
How long it will be before I feel my usual self again	1	2	3	4	5
If there are support groups for people who have had bowel cancer	1	2	3	4	5

Adapted from Graydon et al. (1997)

Communicating information

Detailed advice on multicultural relations, especially related to interpreters and confidentiality

Evidence supports the demand for relevant patient information; however, difficulties have been highlighted when information has been solely reliant on verbal discussion or where language barriers pose a problem. Informal interpreters can cause problems and, because of their lack of clinical knowledge, they may be unreliable (Arif 2003). Family members should not be asked to act as interpreters; it is bad practice and they are likely not to be objective listeners. Organizations should ensure that suitably skilled interpreters and cancer specialists are available for those patients who cannot speak or understand English (DoH 2000, NCGSG 2004, p. 30). Supplementary information in either written or audio-taped format, including language to meet the needs of specific black and ethnic minority groups, is readily available from some cancer charities such as CancerBACUP and Macmillan. Specially prepared literature is available from many NHS hospital departments, individually linked to specific aspects of patient care and patient group. A recognized practice with many cancer departments is audio-taped recording of the interview confirming cancer diagnosis. This means of providing information can be taken away, reviewed and shared with the family at the individual's discretion. Audio or video cassettes are invaluable for those with impaired vision, or hearing or literacy skills. Other requirements to accommodate minority groups include illustrated booklets for learning disability, and interpreters for black and ethnic groups (see Chapter 14).

Creativity is needed to deliver information that is patient centred and provides continuity of care. Health-care policy continues to support the need for interdisciplinary collaboration among professionals. A key development by the Cancer Services Collaborative, to promote equity and consistency of care nationally, is patient information pathways and patient-held records. This represents best practice guidance for the cancer patient and the outcome from its benefit is optimized. As with any form of clinical audit (Figure 8.2), results depend on the reliability of the information collected (Commission for Health Improvement or CHI 2001) (see Chapters 9 and 10).

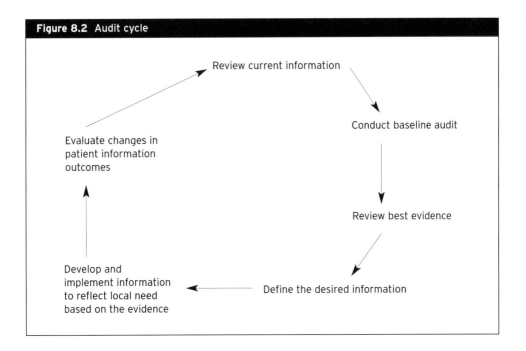

Figure 8.2 Audit cycle

Review current information

Conduct baseline audit

Evaluate changes in patient information outcomes

Review best evidence

Develop and implement information to reflect local need based on the evidence

Define the desired information

Summary of key points

- Assessments should be based on family dynamics, understanding of loss and change, communication and counselling, social policy and resources (see Chapter 14).
- The spiritual dimension of care does not easily lend itself to predicting cause and effect in the emerging need to measure and quantify facets of care and enable the standards of care to be raised. Respecting a patient's religious and spiritual needs does not necessarily imply that action will be taken to meet these needs (DOH 2001).
- Sexual health issues are an important aspect of care. The extent of intervention by health-care staff is determined by many factors including their level of competence,
- Nurses are recognized as key personnel in the NHS modernization programme (DoH 2000) and ideally placed to monitor whether psychological and social care services are responsive to client needs, including those of the carer; because of their own cultural beliefs and practices, they may, however, be unable to respond appropriately. Care enhancement can be successfully achieved only if areas of weakness and concern are highlighted to those responsible for policy implementation.

References

Anon (1976) The PLISSIT model: a proposed conceptual scheme for behavioural treatment of sexual problems. Journal of Sex Education Therapy 2: 1–15.

Arif Z (2003) A different interpretation. Nursing Standard 17: 104.

Barraclough J (1997) Cancer and Emotion: A practical guide to psycho-oncology. New York: John Wiley.

Borwell B (1996) Family under stress. Nursing Times 92(46): 52–3.

Borwell B (1997a) The psychosexual needs of stoma patients. Professional Nurse 12: 250–5.

Borwell B (1997b) Developing Sexual Helping Skills. Maidenhead, Berks: Medical Projects International.

Buckman R (1992) How to Break Bad News: A guide for health-care professionals. London: Papermac.

Cancerlink (1994) Life With Cancer. London: Cancerlink.

Cobbs S (1976) Social support as a moderator of life stress. Psychosomatic Medicine 38: 300–14.

Commission for Health Improvement/Audit Commission (2001) National Service Framework assessments No: 1 NHS cancer care in England and Wales. London: CHI/AC.

Department of Health (2000) The NHS Cancer Plan. London: The Stationery Office.

Department of Health (2001) Your Guide to the NHS: Patient's charter (revised). London: The Stationery Office.

Expert Advisory Group on Cancer (1995) The Calman–Hine Report: A policy framework for commissioning cancer services. London: The Stationery Office.

Fallowfield L (1995) Psychosocial interventions in cancer. British Medical Journal 311: 1316–17.

Fallowfield L, Ford S, Lewis S (1994) Information preferences of patients with cancer. The Lancet 344: 1576.

Fallowfield L, Ratcliffe D, Jenkins V et al. (2000) Psychiatric morbidity and its recognition by doctors in patients with cancer. British Journal of Cancer 84: 1011-15.

Fawzy IF, Fawzy NW, Arndt LA et al. (1995) A critical review of psychosocial interventions in cancer care. Archives of General Psychiatry 52: 100-13 (abstract).

Frude N (1991) Understanding Family Problems: A psychological approach. Chichester: John Wiley.

Graydon J, Palmer-Wickham S, Harrison D et al. (1997) Information needs of women during early treatment for breast cancer. Journal of Advanced Nursing 26: 59-64.

Hart S (1998) Learning-disabled person's experience of general hospitals. British Journal of Nursing 7: 470-7.

Henley A, Schott J (1999) Culture, Religion and Patient Care in a Multi-Ethnic Society. London: Age Concern.

Holmes TH, Rahe RH (1967) The Social Readjustment Scale. Journal of Psychosomatic Research 11: 213-18.

Hopson B (1981) Transition: Understanding and managing personal change. In: Herbert M (ed.), Psychology for Social Workers. London: Macmillan.

Hopwood P, Stephens RJ (2000) Depression in patients with lung cancer: prevalence and risk factors derived from quality of life data. Cited in Fallowfield et al. (2000).

Kasch C (1986) Toward a theory of nursing action: skills and competency in nurse-patient interaction. Nursing Research 35: 226-9.

Krishnasamy M (1996) Social support and the patient with cancer. A review of the literature. Journal of Advanced Nursing 23: 757-62.

Le Var RMH (1998) Improving educational preparation for transcultural health care. Nurse Education Today 18: 519-33.

Macdonald L, Anderson H (1984) Stigma in patients with rectal cancer. Journal of Epidemiology and Health 38: 284-90.

McGreachy C (2001) Spiritual Intelligence in the Workplace. Dublin: Veritas Publishers.

McSherry W, Ross L (2002) Dilemmas of spiritual assessment: considerations for nursing practice. Journal of Advanced Nursing 38: 479-88.

Mills ME, Sullivan K (1999) The importance of information giving for patients newly diagnosed with cancer: a review of the literature. Journal of Clinical Nursing 8: 631-42.

Narayanasamy A (2003) Transcultural nursing: how do nurses respond to cultural needs? British Journal of Nursing 12: 185-94.

National Cancer Guidance Steering Group (2004) Improving Outcomes in Colorectal Cancer: Updated manual. London: NICE.

National Council for Hospices and Specialist Palliative Care Units (2002) Definitions of Supportive and Palliative Care: A consultation paper. London: NCHSPCU.

NHS Executive (1997) Guidance on Commissioning Cancer Services. Improving Outcomes in Colorectal Cancer: The manual. London: HMSO.

Norbeck J (1981) Social support: a model for clinical research and application. Advances in Nursing Science 3(4): 43-59.

Northouse ll (1989) Impact of breast cancer on patients and husbands. Cancer Nursing 12: 276-84.

Parkes CM (1993) Bereavement as a psychosocial transition. In: Stroebe MS, Stroebe W, Hanson RO (eds), Handbook of Bereavement. Cambridge: Cambridge University Press.

Price B (1998) Cancer: altered body image. Nursing Standard 12(21): 49-55.

Roberts D, Snowball J (1999) Psychosocial care in oncology nursing: a study of social knowledge. Journal of Clinical Nursing 8: 39-47.

Royal College of Nursing (2000) Sexuality and Sexual Health. London: RCN.

Sheldon F (1997) Psychosocial Palliative Care. Cheltenham: Stanley Thornes.

Shell JA, Kirsch S (2001) Psychosocial issues, outcomes and quality of life. In: Otto SE (ed.), Oncology Nursing. 4th edn. St Louis, MI: Mosby Inc.

Shontz F (1975) The Psychological Aspects of Physical Illness. New York: Macmillan

Stoter D (2002) Spiritual Pain. In: Penson J, Fisher RA (eds) Palliative Care for People With Cancer, 3rd edn. London: Arnold.

Taylor EJ (1993) Factors associated with meaning in life among people with recurrent cancer. Oncology Nursing Forum 20: 1399–405.

Williams HA (1986) Nurses attitudes towards sexuality in cancer patients. Oncology Nursing Forum 13(2): 39–43.

Woods NF, Lamb MA (1981) Sexuality and the cancer patient. Cancer Nursing 4: 137–44.

Further reading

Barraclough J (1997) Cancer and Emotion: A practical guide to psycho-oncology. New York: J Wiley.

Henley A, Schott J (1999) Culture, Religion and Patient Care in a Multi-Ethnic Society: A handbook for professionals. London: Age Concern.

Lloyd-Williams M (ed.) (2003) Psychosocial Issues in Palliative Care. Oxford: Oxford University Press.

Chapter 9

Promoting a patient-centred approach to care

Barbara Borwell

A person may be identified as having colorectal/bowel cancer in many ways, and after diagnosis management of the disease relies on several issues and agencies to support the efficacy and equity of care.

In 1998 the Department of Health (DoH) adopted the principles of best practice guidelines in order to ensure that treatment was delivered to patients by clinicians who were specialists in that field, avoiding local variation in health-care provision. At the same time the National Institute for Clinical Excellence (NICE) was established to evaluate the evidence, based on clinical efficacy and cost-effectiveness, of a range of interventions, including treatments and technology. NICE is also responsible for the development of clinical guidelines relating to a specific condition such as cancer (NICE 2003); however, they do recognize the importance of responding to individual need and priorities. Key government documents consistently identify cancer as a national priority and recommend a programme of specific reforms in the delivery of cancer services (DoH 1997, 2003).

The organization of care through multidisciplinary treatment and support teams specializing in specific aspects of the cancer journey is seen as important for optimal care and improved outcome, based on nationally agreed protocols (National Cancer Guidance Steering Group or NCGSG 2004) (Figure 9.1 and see Chapter 1).

Team structure

Recommendations for a colorectal cancer multidisciplinary team (MDT) to take responsibility for this group of patients is clearly defined in the revised *Improving Outcomes in Colorectal Cancer* document (NCGSG 2004). Cancer networks are now responsible for the specialization of membership criteria of these teams in general hospitals versus the specialist cancer centre, and reflect the provision of treatment and care required throughout the cancer journey.

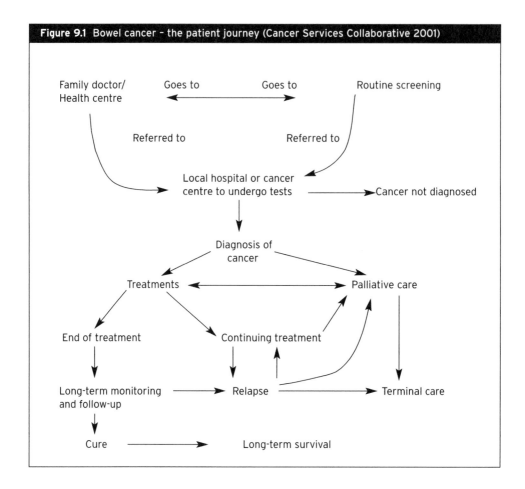

Figure 9.1 Bowel cancer – the patient journey (Cancer Services Collaborative 2001)

Core team

The core team consists of the following:

- Surgeons (minimum of two): specialists in colorectal cancer or with established interest and expertise in colorectal cancer techniques (NCGSG 2004)
- Oncologist with a special interest in bowel cancer, either a clinical oncologist who is able to provide chemotherapy and radiotherapy or a medical oncologist collaborating with the radiotherapy centre
- Gastroenterologist
- Histopathologist
- Diagnostic radiologist with gastrointestinal expertise
- Skilled colonoscopist from any discipline: surgeon, physician or specialist nurse
- Specialist nurses including stoma and colorectal nurses
- Meeting coordinator/team secretary.

MDTs (Figure 9.2) should remain in close contact with other health professionals (HPs) who may be co-opted as part of an extended team such as general practitioner and primary health-care team, specialist palliative care teams, dietitian, geneticist, counsellor, psychologist, liver/thoracic surgeons, social worker, clinical trials coordinator. Anal cancer MDTs should be based in cancer centres to provide treatment for these patients. Allied professionals are appointed as appropriate, e.g. physiotherapist or occupational therapist for individual needs.

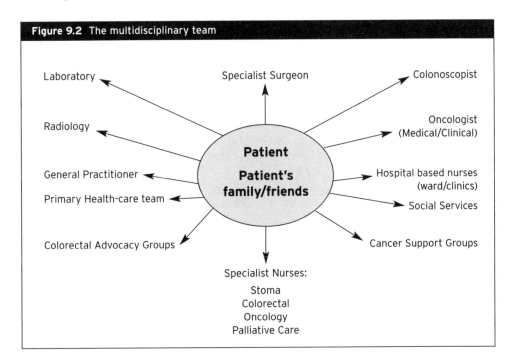

Figure 9.2 The multidisciplinary team

The provision of high-class seamless care and patient support, with cost reductions and improved clinical effectiveness, has placed additional pressure on service providers. Integrated care pathways (ICPs), also referred to as care maps/critical/clinical pathways, set out best practice guidance and predict the course of events for a specific group of patients. These are specified on a time frame, with incidents, actions and interventions identified by designated health professionals. Care pathways are multidisciplinary plans of recorded care, forming all or part of the clinical record, providing documentation of the care given and thus facilitating the evaluation of outcomes. The analysis of what actual care has taken place highlights areas for improving the quality of care, e.g. delayed discharge (see earlier), which are developed in response to the demand to define clinical services and foster partnerships with other organizations. Encompassed within the clinical governance framework, they act as an audit tool to monitor any digression or variation from the expected plan of care.

High-quality nursing and supportive care is usually an expectation of patients. This quality tool, suitably applied, with clearly defined, locally agreed, outcome-based treatment goals, has the ability to deliver effective patient-centred care; if used inappropriately its effectiveness will be greatly reduced.

Criticisms of ICPs (Figure 9.3) argue that they ignore personalized care, reflecting the traditional medical model, which is oriented towards the disease/cure route (Hunter 1995). However, the pathways are a concept rather than being concrete, and are potentially flexible, allowing modification by the HP. Individual needs not covered in the pathway can be highlighted and allowances made. Successful pathway development relies on involvement of an interdisciplinary team with members designated to look at specific aspects of care to ascertain where improvements can be made. They are seen as more effective when there is a predictable course of care or procedure such as surgery/treatment for colorectal cancer. Specific aspects of care can be monitored based on agreed standards of best practice such as preoperative preparation, reflecting local practice of all those involved in caring for the patient at this phase of the journey, including allied HPs.

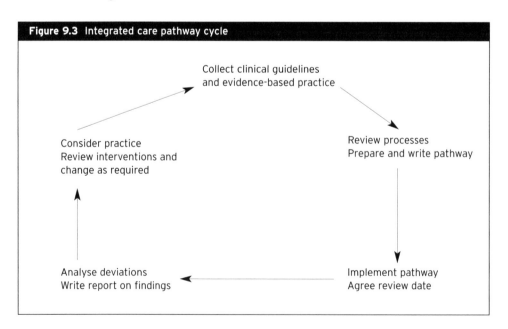

Figure 9.3 Integrated care pathway cycle

Collect clinical guidelines
and evidence-based practice

Consider practice
Review interventions and
change as required

Review processes
Prepare and write pathway

Analyse deviations
Write report on findings

Implement pathway
Agree review date

Indications suggest that this method can increase patient satisfaction, through enhanced communication and collaboration between MDT members, promote best practice and reduce the period of hospitalization, without increasing the risk of problems (Guezo 2003).

Assessment

The quality of care is essentially a matter of values and measurement. As the health service becomes more resource minded, HPs need to make sure that quality is their prime objective. The biographical and general health data gained at the initial interview form the basis of assessment. This profile allows other health-related issues or concerns to be reviewed and identified (Figure 9.4).

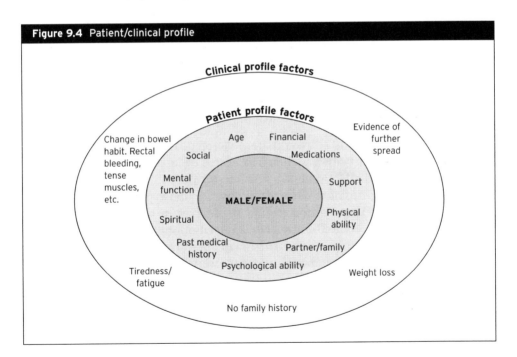

Figure 9.4 Patient/clinical profile

Clinical assessment

The health history varies according to the patient's current health problem. An outline assessment at this stage, conducted by the GP and based on specified Department of Health guidelines, establishes the priority of investigations such as rectal bleeding, and suspected cancer indicates referral to a colorectal clinic within 2 weeks (www.doh.gov.uk/cancer). The GP is the gatekeeper in the referral of cancer patients, in spite of organizational changes and access to specialized care by other means. Some trusts have established a standard referral proforma to improve this process (NCGSG 2004).

A detailed clinical assessment based on current and relevant past history, written in a chronological manner, provides a contextual account of the development of symptoms from the patient's perspective. This includes patient opinion and thoughts about the symptoms, and their effect on daily life, function and significance. In some instances a family member, or friend, may have prompted referral. Most colorectal departments use systematic, coded, data collection sheets, which offer consistency, facility for audit and potential research information. Information acquired at this stage allows an action plan to be negotiated, which could include further diagnostic tests, treatment and evaluation. Effective communication, patient involvement and understanding throughout this process are essential. Additional supportive information may be required to reinforce what has been discussed.

Communication and information

In the current health-care climate it is accepted that limited time will be available to talk with patients. The centre of attention must therefore be on quality and effectiveness of the interaction.

Receiving a diagnosis of cancer is, for most patients, a frightening experience. Patients suddenly find themselves in a threatening environment with little time to comprehend and emotionally adjust to the turmoil of decision-making about treatment options. Communicating with patients is a topic commonly under scrutiny and the focus of many studies (Edwards and Miller 2001, Isaksen et al. 2003). The way in which information is communicated and the use of appropriate language can have a powerful and lasting effect on patients. The choice of words can potentially confuse, frighten and intimidate (Buggins 1995). Links between understanding the communication process and patients' subsequent satisfaction and compliance have also been considered (Ley 1995). The nature of nursing places the nurse in a privileged position to communicate on a one-to-one basis while undertaking necessary procedures, to verify understanding and identify particular concerns.

Effective communication channels between the MDT and patients and significant others, built on understanding and mutual trust, are essential, and include the GP; these channels should be used for information about the diagnosis, treatment and potential outcome. Patients frequently contact their GPs to discuss their treatment options, and it is paramount that details of information discussed at consultation and throughout the phases of the cancer journey be conveyed to them.

Empowering patients through information about their health-care options is seen as a government priority (DoH 2000a), including the recruitment of patients into clinical trials for newer treatment modalities and evaluation of their efficiency. Better dissemination of information about the relevance of well-designed clinical trials for the development of quality cancer care is needed for both patients and the community.

Today, information is widely sought on every topic, verified by the enthusiastic response to the internet. Patients seek information for a variety of reasons. Irrespective of their disease, relevant information, whether good or bad, is recognized as a coping mechanism for a change in health status, to assist with the adaptation to the uncertainties inherent in cancer (Graydon et al. 1997; see also Chapter 8). Health professionals acknowledge these facts and yet cancer patients still report a lack of information about their condition (Coulter et al. 1999). *The National Cancer Plan* specifies a maximum 2-week wait for those suspected of having cancer. Other directives include the benefit of pre-planned and pre-booked care by 2004 (DoH 2000b). Patient education material, via written information, to promote understanding about their care in preparation for clinic attendance or pre-clinic investigations, leading to diagnosis and treatment such as colonoscopy, needs to be sent out with these appointments.

There is a fundamental need for quality information from the providers of health services that ensures respect for cultural diversity. Information about colorectal cancer and its management is given in many ways and the language must reflect the range of ethnic communities, and can be verbal, written, visual or pre-recorded to support or supplement oral communication. 'Virtual understanding' is a recently launched website to help ease the anxiety and demystify the experience of visiting a cancer clinic (Royal College of Radiologists 2003). With advanced technology and expertise, the period of hospitalization is now greatly reduced, and the demand for written information is mounting.

Written material supports verbal information. The design and presentation are important, and developed from a patient perspective. User involvement in health care, which acknowledges the patients' needs and experiences, can increase satisfaction and enhance patient empowerment (Entwhistle et al. 1997, Coulter et al. 1999). Empowerment seeks to recognize the power that exists between the HP and patient, enabling partnerships to be established while appreciating a patient's own inner resources in the decision-making process (Grahn 1996).

The establishment of specialist teams and nurses for site-specific cancers such as colorectal cancer, and for stoma care, seeks to improve information, support and care throughout the cancer journey (DoH 2000a). In-house information and patient-held diaries are now familiar in most centres, providing details of the care pathway and those responsible for specific aspects of care. Consequential to treatment are changes related to self-concept and body image. The specialist team have a responsibility to help the patient clarify his or her situation and values, to ensure that decision-making is based on personal goals and desires. This is demonstrated by Soloman et al.'s (2003) study, which compared 'acting patient surrogacy by clinicians' with patient preferences. Disparity was found between the clinicians' decision when acting on their behalf and patients' decisions when they were able to trade off survival for quality of life. Recording of patient preferences through scenarios indicated that patients were generally opposed to chemotherapy, inclining towards surgery with a permanent colostomy. This emphasizes the need for partnership between HPs and patients in the decision-making process.

Improving the quality of life for cancer patients and their families by the provision of timely and adequate information and education is an important part of the nurses' role. The Nursing and Midwifery Council's (NMC's) Code of Conduct denotes respect for patient autonomy and 'their right to decide whether or not to undergo any health intervention' (NMC 2002, clause 3.2) (see Chapter 12). There is a lack of awareness, from the public viewpoint, that nurses are a significant source of cancer information and education. The provision of information is seen as descriptive and explanatory in a one-way communication, whereas education is a more interactive process based on learning theories and dispensing information, with the aim of holistically changing the way patients think, feel and behave with respect to the proposed treatment for colorectal cancer and to engage them actively in their rehabilitation (Grahn 1996). Patient satisfaction is rated higher for those with access to a clinical nurse specialist (CNS) (Mills and Sullivan 1999).

Nursing assessment

The nursing contribution to society is concerned with meeting the needs of the person, the family and the community, based on the best available evidence for a specific aspect of patient care. Patient-centred care relies on needs being effectively met and a responsibility for nurses to treat each individual uniquely. The goal of nursing as a moral practice is supposedly 'good care'; often, purposeful work in nursing is outside traditional nursing values, governed by cost-effectiveness and shorter hospital stay. Inadequate fulfilment of health-care needs can restrict a person's ability to achieve his or her full potential. Assessment acts as a basis for all other phases of health and well-being. Without effective assessment, good quality care planning is unattainable (Crossfield 1989).

The quality of assessment is variable. Related attributes include practitioner competency in interviewing, communication and social skills. Getting to know the patient well and establishing a good therapeutic nurse–patient relationship is essential in cancer nursing. Patients visit frequently for months or years as they return for treatment and surveillance appointments. For reliability, assessment information should be based around a conceptual framework, to consolidate and signify the holistic nature of caring (Crossfield 1989). This systematic approach to developing the scientific body of knowledge within nursing serves to support the contribution of a professional service to society and a foundation for nursing practice. A nursing model identifies and represents the essential concepts or elements of nursing. Nursing theorists' approach towards the development and use of nursing models is not dissimilar but does imply a different focus on how the main elements of nursing are addressed.

It is not the intention of this chapter to provide broad details of nursing theory, but examples based on Orem's (1991) self-care model are applied for the patient with colorectal cancer (Table 9.1). This model has three related parts:

1. Deficit in self-care, when an individual is unable to meet the demands of self-care as a result of their ability, either health derived or health related, and to predict nursing requirement.

2. Self-care as a deliberate action learned from contact and communication, functioning as an integrated whole, self-reliant on individual beliefs and knowledge about health care, including the well-being of dependants. This is influenced by cultural and social experiences throughout the life cycle. Self-care agents include: self, parent, relative, nurse or carer. Orem (1991) acknowledges that certain humanistic needs or self-care requirements are necessary to support the balance between health and illness comprising sufficient:
   (a) intake of air
   (b) intake of water
   (c) intake of food
   (d) elimination
   (e) activity and rest

(f) social interaction and solitude

(g) prevention of hazards

(h) promotion of human functioning and development

(i) development of self-care requisites relating to life changes

3. Health deviation, arising from ill-health and demanding a change in self-care behaviour.

Table 9.1 Preoperative nursing assessment based on Orem's theory

a. **Assessing the patient with colorectal cancer**
   For surgery and formation of stoma
   Nursing process (assess–plan–implement–evaluate–review)
   Theoretical framework
   Questioning and observation

b. **Questioning: general**
   History
   Symptoms: when, duration, severity, stable/unstable?
   Onset: sudden or gradual?
   Influencing factors?
   What gives relief from the symptoms?

c. **Questioning: specific**
   Physical/mental abilities?
   Attitudes towards stoma?
   Nutrition, diet, medication?
   Nature of lifestyle activities?
   Previous knowledge/type of stoma?
   Skin: any existing/history of skin problems?
   Environment: toilet facilities?
   Understanding of condition/treatment?
   Employment/financial status?
   Relationships: existing, nature?
   Sexuality: homosexual/heterosexual?

d. **Observations**
   Physique/stature
   Skin texture, colour/condition
   Body contours, scars, bony prominences
   Skin colour (lips, nose, ear lobes, mouth)
   Alertness and orientation
   Activity tolerance
   Integration/communication with others

e. **Nursing diagnoses**
   Patient to have abdominoperineal excision of the rectum (APER) and permanent colostomy
   Partner reluctant to be involved
   Skin sensitive to adhesive tape
   Activity intolerance, fatigue
   Fear, anxiety, powerlessness

Table 9.1 Preoperative nursing assessment based on Orem's theory contd'

Sleep pattern disturbance
Social isolation
Risk of infection/complications

f. Nursing interventions
Contact stoma care nurse
Counselling
Offer patient information/resources
Ensure toilet accessible
Support/reassure patient/partner
Pharmacological interventions: aperients, wash-outs
Commence low-residue diet/oral fluids 24 hrs before surgery.

g. Facilitating adaptation/self-care/health promotion
Strategies for maintaining independence
Toilet: accessible/commode
Encourage mobility
Introduce to other patients, offer visitor from ostomy association
Counselling, support, discussion/exploration
Ability to attain self-care
Demonstrate suitable stoma pouch

h. Orem's nursing systems (example) (supportive/educative)
Patient's role
Meet self-care requirements
Continue to learn and develop self-care abilities
Nursing role
Assist patients with decision-making, e.g. surgery, stoma site
Facilitate patient learning about: stoma, self-care skills, assess/demonstrate appropriate
stoma pouch, access to problem-solving network, update information regularly

From Cavanagh (1991)

Current and future self-care ability is calculated to establish what the patient normally achieves when functioning in his or her usual capacity. It is determined from the present state of health, possibly compromised by disease, and the potential ability after medical intervention, e.g. abdominal surgery. An existing health deficit such as visual impairment may have a future influence on self-care ability after the stoma formation.

The nursing diagnosis determines whether a person can be helped through planned nursing action. Cavanagh (1991, p. 24) discusses actions undertaken by nurses to enable patients to achieve specific health goals. To fulfil this obligation, certain requisites are necessary, which include generating a strategy for nursing interaction, and establishing the ratio between the nurse–patient contribution of self-care demands and adequate resources to meet these actions. Cavanagh (1991) explains that these needs create a nursing system to assist a person through nursing intervention. The elements essential to nursing include:

- assisting, helping and intervening
- nurses who are knowledgeable, capable and skilful
- people receiving care
- results of nursing actions.

Care is seen as health (universal), developmental and illness (health deviation) dimensions. Individuals therefore perform universal (health) self-care, developmental self-care and health deviation (illness) self-care. Individuals able to manage their own self-care can:

- support essential physical, psychological and social life processes
- maintain human structure and functions
- develop their human potential to its maximum
- prevent injury or disease
- cure or regulate disease (with appropriate assistance)
- cure or regulate the effects of disease (with appropriate assistance).

Changes that can affect the balance of the life cycle, causing a self-care deficit include the following:

- Poor health/disability
- Oppressive living conditions
- Status issues, social or economic
- Social adaptation
- Bereavement: sudden or expected of close relative/friends
- Educational deprivation
- Loss of job/possessions.

Nursing goals

- Meet the deficit until the patient is able to meet it him- or herself or meet the total need
- Enable the patient to increase his or her ability to meet the demand
- Enable the patient's relative/significant other to meet the demand
- Meet the total need.

Nursing systems for care delivery to meet the self-care deficit exist at three levels: totally compensatory, partly compensatory and educative/supportive.

Totally compensatory

Patient role
The patient is totally dependent for all his or her self-care needs.

Nursing role

Wholly compensating for self-care inabilities, providing support and guidance, making clinical judgements based on patient need, acting as the patient's advocate in decision-making, and empowering the patient by cultivating existing skills.

Partly compensatory

Patient role

Performs some self-care activities with assistance from nursing staff.

Nursing role

Completing self-care activities for the patient to compensate for any limitations, providing assistance as needed.

Educative/supportive

Nursing care is delivered by:

- recognising and addressing the patient's needs
- teaching
- guiding
- supporting the patient, physically and psychologically
- providing and maintaining a safe environment.

Nursing management and care

Many hospitals and specialist colorectal departments have developed guidelines and standards to optimize care for patients undergoing treatment for colorectal cancer. The Royal College of Nursing (RCN 2002), and specialist nurse representatives from the Gastroenterology and Stoma Care Nursing Forum, have developed competencies to help nurses caring for patients with colorectal problems achieve a minimal level of care. Nurses working in specialized roles require additional knowledge and skills to ensure that effectual and evidence-based care is delivered. Used with locally produced guidelines and in conjunction with ICPs these offer a standardized measurable package of care (RCN 2002). Patients, however, have individual, variable needs and expectations of nursing care. Unless nurses acknowledge these perceptions and allocate time to listening and caring, the patients' experience of care is more likely to have a negative response.

Preoperative considerations

Patients diagnosed with colorectal cancer will have undergone a period of anxiety and uncertainty while awaiting investigation results. Finally they are informed about the need for elective surgery, which may be curative; with additional treatment their chance of survival could be increased or their treatment will be palliative in advanced disease. Personality, cultural and religious beliefs, body image and social stigma are issues that need sensitive assessment. (Surgery requiring a stoma has additional considerations and is discussed separately. However, many of the principles relating to nursing care and management are applicable to all patients with colorectal cancer.)

Information given preoperatively is unlikely to be retained and individual reactions are variable (see Chapter 8). Many patients prefer to talk through their concerns before being admitted into hospital. Contact details of appropriate people including the GP and a CNS such as a colorectal or stoma nurse should be given. Where a patient-held diary is used these details are documented. Providing appropriate information can empower patients to seek further details, and act as a trigger for future questions, reinforcing discussion or clarification before giving consent for the proposed operation (see Chapter 5). Specifically focused information is particularly significant and can facilitate psychological adaptation (National Cancer Alliance 1996).

Preparation for surgery should consider all essential health-care requisites: age, culture, religion and spirituality, and the potential effect on individuals and their families physically, emotionally and psychologically. The alleviation of anxieties through the provision of appropriate information and discussion aids rehabilitation (Kelly 1992).

Establishing a patient's immediate postoperative expectations, and enabling him or her to express his or her fears, misconceptions and concerns about the anticipated recovery, can facilitate this process. After curative surgery patients can encounter disease-linked problems that affect their quality of life (Sprangers et al. 1995). Functions such as eating, drinking and elimination may be significantly disrupted (see Chapter 5). Patients requiring stoma formation are more likely to experience additional problems concerning body image and sexuality.

Other influences on postoperative recovery

Nutritional support may be required preoperatively and/or postoperatively to attain repletion in those at increased risk (see Chapter 11). Diagnostic symptoms, such as physical weakness caused by poor nutritional status, put patients in danger of developing postoperative malnutrition, with delayed recovery in, for example, wound healing. Psychosocial issues can have similar consequences – typically avoidance of certain foods, where patients have manipulated their diet to evade embarrassing situations or withdrawn from social activities.

Specific considerations for stoma surgery

Preoperative

Preparation includes physical, psychological and social factors; for maximization of care a structured approach is required (Table 9.1; see also Chapter 5).

After the decision that surgery will entail formation of a stoma, either temporary or permanent, a member of the colorectal team should alert the stoma care nurse, preferably at the time of the outpatient consultation to enable the nurse to understand the details given to the patient by the surgeon. Maintenance of consistency of information forms a basis for further discussions between the patient and the family. Establishment of an early trusting relationship is essential, especially when surgery is palliative. Acknowledging the patient preference, a further pre-admission appointment should be made, ideally in a hospital quiet room or in the patient's home, based on available resources and service provision. Studies demonstrate the value of preoperative information and discussion helps to alleviate anxiety, particularly in the time lapse between diagnosis and admission into hospital (McCahon 1999). Anxiety can be portrayed in many ways and at varying levels; some patients may appear indifferent to discussing surgery but this does not signify that the information is not required (Borwell 1997). Giving patients an opportunity to verbalize their fears and concerns enables them to develop their coping mechanisms. Literature specific to the type of operation, with diagrams of the gastrointestinal system, stoma and pouching systems, should be offered.

Preoperative assessment by the stoma care or experienced nurse is essential for successful rehabilitation and discharge preparation. Significant factors include stoma siting, mental and physical abilities, manual dexterity, lifestyle and predisposing skin conditions to determine the most suitable appliance type (Table 9.2). A poorly sited stoma leads to future difficulties in stoma management. This procedure usually takes place the day before surgery, with the patient's consent and participation (see Chapter 5). Some patients, at this stage, may cope by distancing themselves from their body. Patient involvement is vital for ethical and practical reasons; facilitating empowerment through ownership of the body and the stoma can help psychological adaptation. The wearing of a typical stoma pouch preoperatively can also aid this process.

Table 9.2 Appliance assessment guidelines

Assessment	Problem	Goal	Action
1. Physique	Stature Weight Contours	Appliance to be comfortable and mould to body contours	Ostomy pouches available in range of lengths/shape, e.g. standard/small Flange soft and flexible, rigid or convex
2. Mental ability	Age Intelligence	Simplicity	Acquisition of new skills can be difficult
3. Physical ability and manual dexterity	Disability, e.g. paraplegia Capability, e.g. arthritis	Promote patient independence	May need assistance with stoma care
4. Shape, size, stoma site	Badly sited stoma Irregular shape Large/small	Appliance security Appliance to fit snugly around base of stoma	Ensure flat surface for appliance adhesion Cut-to-fit appliances will accommodate shape of stoma Measure stoma correctly using a template; allow 3 mm clearance.
5. Skin	Previous skin condition, e.g. psoriasis Sensitive skin	Minimize trauma Maintain security and dignity	Patch test before surgery Use hypoallergenic adhesive Two-piece appliance with integral skin protective wafer Skin care aids, e.g. lotions, barrier film
6. Type of stoma	Consistency of effluent, soft, firm, liquid Frequency of action Flatus	Knowledge and understanding of surgery	Closed-end appliance; less than two pouches daily or two-piece system Drainable, open-ended device May require dietary advice or medication to regulate bowel action Consider pouch with integral charcoal filter
7. Nature of lifestyle	Mobility Social Financial Individual needs	Preoperative siting of stoma, to minimize interference with usual lifestyle Promote rehabilitation	Range of appliances available to enable individual needs to be met Ensure patient awareness of prescription exemption costs if permanent stoma

Postoperative considerations

Postoperatively the stoma care nurse works with the MDT (see Figure 9.2, p. 149) providing specific stoma care guidance and coordinating patient education in preparation for discharge. Care will be the same as for anyone undergoing major abdominal surgery; in addition observation and monitoring of the stoma are required.

Patient education and teaching

Awareness should be raised about patient expectations after surgery, particularly anticipated operation outcomes, intravenous therapy, pain control, dressings, wound drains, stoma appearance and output. In the perioperative period a viable stoma is moist, usually shiny red in colour, and swollen as a result of postoperative oedema. Early complications may include the following:

- Ischaemia caused by vascular insufficiency with subsequent retraction and stenosis, with possible immediate surgical revision.
- Mucocutaneous separation where the suture line is interrupted at the mucocutaneous junction, forming a cavity at the area of stoma disconnection. This can be distressing for the patient with potential appliance leakage, presenting challenges for stoma care management (Boyd-Carson et al. 2004) (Table 9.3).

Table 9.3 Postoperative stoma care monitoring record

Stoma care nurse:				Sited by:			
Date of operation:							
Type of operation:							
Specific instructions:				Sited by:			
				Bridge *in situ*		Yes/No	
				Remove:		Date	
				Removed by:		Date	
Appearance of stoma and skin							
Date	Time	Colour	Oedema	Protruding or flush	Skin		Signature
Stoma output							
Date	Time	Colour	Fluid	Formed	Constipated		Signature

To facilitate easy observation a clear open-ended pouch is worn. Once bowel function is restored the initial output can be quite offensive. This is normal as a result of the collection of intestinal gases and fasting, but gradually subsides once nutritional intake is recommenced.

Accomplishing self-care skills and becoming totally responsible for stoma care management can be daunting for patients and carers. The care plan should include goals for self-care in preparation for discharge, based on information obtained at the core assessment (see Table 9.1).

Successful teaching is reliant on establishing learning needs, including those of the carer where achievement of stoma care management relies on his or her involvement. Skill acquisition depends on cognitive and psychomotor ability, correctly demonstrating the procedure as a whole and divided into manageable parts. Setting small realistic goals and working at an individual level and pace has many benefits (McCahon 1999, p. 178):

1. Achievement of each stage gives patient satisfaction
2. Ongoing motivating factor
3. Level of independence is measurable.

The earlier self-care is taught, the sooner dignity and self-esteem are restored.

Appliances and skin care

Effective stoma management involves the following:

- An appliance-selection criterion and skin care regimen to reflect individual needs
- Ascertaining a system for changing, emptying, disposal and obtaining future supplies
- Collaborative approach to patient education
- Regular assessment, e.g. body contour changes caused by medication or progressive disease
- Consideration of circumstances that pre-empt stoma surgery, e.g. a palliative procedure.

Selection of an appropriate pouching system

Advances in technology have resulted in the availability of an extensive range of high-quality products within western society, allowing individual requirements to be accommodated. An essential part of the stoma care nurse's role is to ensure that pouching systems are secure, thereby helping patients to feel confident and resume social activities (Mckenzie and Ingram 2001). The pouches are made of odour-proof, clear or opaque, flexible plastic, with either a closed or an open end to allow emptying which is secured with a closing device. Appliances may be a one-piece system with a base plate (flange) combined, or two-piece systems with a separate flange and pouch connected by a variety of techniques. Flatus filters, integral to most closed pouches, are optional on some drainable types. Correctly fitted, appliances should fit snugly around the stoma base allowing a 2–3 mm clearance. To minimize pouch leakage and skin problems regular measurement using a measuring guide is essential (see Table 9.2).

Additional considerations in stoma care

Emergency surgery

As a result of the nature of their physical and acute medical condition, patients requiring emergency surgery lack the preparation before and period of adjustment to diagnosis and surgery. These patients may be at increased risk of psychological problems, which can affect ways of coping and rehabilitation. Additional sympathetic support at the time of surgery, and thereafter involving close family support, can help alleviate such problems and patient maintenance.

Effects of stoma on sexuality and body image

Psychological support is ongoing, mindful that after colorectal cancer surgery, whether sphincter saving or sphincter sacrificing, a patient's bowel or sexual function may be compromised (Sprangers et al. 1995). At this stage patients are most vulnerable when coping strategies are depleted; the implications of surgical mutilation are apparent, including transient losses related to self-care and independence. Nursing support should focus on raising confidence and self-esteem, acknowledging anxieties and offering reassurance, with emphasis on what patients can accomplish. Addressing issues, such as stained bedding or clothing, assistance with personal hygiene, showing compassionate respect for the finer details, is important. Equally significant is diligence over stoma care technique. The patient concern is centred on odour and pouches. Leakage is demoralizing, and will destroy dignity and provoke negative thoughts about the future. Postoperatively, psychological and sexual support should concur with patient teaching, sensitively encouraging observation and involvement, reflecting on information given preoperatively and the position of the stoma on the body. At this time patients are receptive to verbal and non-verbal reactions from staff and visitors. Adjusting to the consequences of surgery with changes in body image and function is a major life event (see Chapter 8). The following is a useful guide.

Psychological recovery milestones

- Begins to look at and touch stoma
- Allows others to look
- Expresses interest, asking questions about caring for the stoma
- Begins to take over responsibility for stoma care
- Socializes with patients and visitors.

Patients undergoing stoma formation face permanent changes to their accepted body image, lifestyle and sexuality. Changes affecting physical appearance can involve a sense of loss that can be experienced in many ways. Patients feel less appealing as a result of their changed body shape and functioning stoma, and doubt their ability to continue everyday existence. There are many aspects to adjustment; patients must learn to care for their stoma and restore themselves into society to an acceptable level. In time most people adapt and cope well with their stoma because of a natural mental healing process. Some patients may find this adaptation process too complicated and require specialist help in coming to terms with the impact of diagnosis and surgery.

Impairment of sexual function is consistently prevalent among those with sphincter-sacrificing surgery (see Chapter 5), irrespective of gender and sexual orientation, and often connected to anxieties about partner rejection and failure. Reports indicate that stoma and non-stoma patients have limitations in the level of social functioning, especially those with a colostomy (Sprangers et al. 1995, p. 361). Practical suggestions could incorporate ways to enhance personal appearance and appeal to a partner, subsequently enhancing a person's confidence and self-esteem. Achieving this for a woman could include attractive lingerie, disguising the stoma pouch with a pretty cover and wearing a smaller pouch for discreetness. Enhancing bodily presentation in the male is equally important. Promoting pouch security, thus reducing the stress and embarrassment of pouch leakage, by ensuring an empty pouch before love making is important (Borwell 1999) (see Chapter 8).

Ageing

Colorectal cancer affects mainly older people. Information retention and skill acquisition can diminish with age, and any existing debilitating medical condition may cause impaired vision and less manual dexterity. Adverse effects of medication prescribed to treat some disorders, e.g. corticosteroids, may affect skin integrity. Concerns about future independence on discharge may be a problem for any patient with an established physical, mental or medical disorder. It is important to reassure the patient and significant carer about the teaching of self-care skills and support to conserve independence on discharge.

Culture

Cultural and religious beliefs and personal requirements, including patient values and attitudes towards their condition, are particularly pertinent to bowel surgery and stoma formation. Some patients may keep to a modesty code, which restrains them from touch or body exposure, especially by someone of the opposite sex. Approaches to personal hygiene and anal management may also differ, where personal cleanliness is linked to spiritual purity. Nurses should be sensitive to these needs and attempt to observe the distress that this may cause to both the patient and the family (Henley and Schott 1999).

Side effects of treatment

Management of colorectal cancer often requires an approach using multiple methods, where treatments need particular care and surveillance. Patients requiring radiotherapy and chemotherapy are likely to undergo further physiological and psychosocial changes as a result of their toxicity. In addition, those patients who have a stoma may experience alteration to the appearance, size, shape and function of the stoma. Regular surveillance may be necessary throughout treatment to detect early stoma-related problems.

Radiotherapy (see Chapter 7)

The field of treatment is usually planned to avoid or reduce irradiation damage in the stomal area by decreasing the doses. In some instances the tumour to be irradiated is deeply situated behind the stoma and problems can occur. Pouching systems today are generally manufactured using synthetic materials; where metallic components are included their use should be discontinued for the period of treatment. Colostomy irrigation, if used, should also be discontinued. Patient information should include the effects of acute irradiation damage on the gastrointestinal system and the impact on stomal function, and on the skin and mucosa. A review of current management routine could prevent future skin problems, e.g. replacing a closed pouch with a drainable one that is more appropriate for a liquid stool. Regular monitoring of the size, shape and condition of the stoma is essential (see Tables 9.2 and 9.3). Gentle cleansing with warm water can alleviate stoma ulceration, and drying with a soft tissue, and then applying a special barrier powder such as Orahesive, will allow adherence to moist mucous membranes. A two-piece pouching system allows frequent attention without increasing the risk of skin trauma resulting from frequent pouch changes.

Increases in stoma output require patient monitoring for signs of dehydration, the ileostomy patient being particularly vulnerable. Observe for signs of electrolyte disturbance, such as confusion and dry skin. Dietary advice to extend the transit time, including the reduction of high fibre-based foods (see Chapter 11), and anti-diarrhoeal drugs to decrease the volume and replacement of fluid and electrolyte loss, may be necessary.

Chemotherapy (see Chapter 6)

General awareness and management of the side effects of chemotherapeutic agents on the gastrointestinal system apply, in addition to the following.

Diarrhoea

Management is the same as discussed for radiotherapy; the appliance should be checked for security and emptied before the pouch becomes half-full.

Paralytic ileus or constipation

When paralytic ileus occurs oral intake is discontinued and replaced by other routes. Constipation, only a potential problem for the person with a colostomy, will require increased amounts of fluids and roughage.

Peripheral neuropathy and neurotoxicity

Manual dexterity can be impaired and may affect patient independence; a review of current pouching system or involvement of other carers may be required.

Myelosuppression

Observe and promote careful peristomal skin care routine and swab for potential infection. Advice includes minimizing the risk of trauma; skin shaving around the peristomal area should be discontinued until after treatment, and vigorous cleansing and drying avoided. The prevalence of infection and trauma is related to patient technique, changes in skin permeability caused by medication or treatments, and any coexisting skin problems such as psoriasis and folliculitis, commonly found in men who need to remove body hair around the stoma. The presence of infection needs medical advice; however, treatment of skin or fungal infections can affect pouch adhesion and security. The use of an occlusive dressing on to which the appliance is attached can usually resolve this problem.

Patient information literature available from national charitable organizations such as CancerBACUP (see Chapter 14) or developed by local cancer centres offers guidance and can assist in the reinforcement of verbal information.

Palliative care (see Chapter 10)

The nature of palliative surgery suggests that removal of tumour aims not to cure but to relieve symptoms that are tumour related. Ongoing bowel obstruction caused by the tumour may be either relieved or minimized (Breckman 1998). Additional treatments such as radiotherapy, laser or chemotherapy may be offered as adjuvant therapy to palliative surgery and, as previously discussed, are not without problems, particularly for those with a stoma. In addition, the context in which surgery was performed may now be affected by other palliative interventions for a pre-terminal or terminal condition.

Stoma surgery is used as a palliative procedure, when patients:

- have an existing stoma for colorectal cancer, which was potentially curative, but develop local recurrent or distant metastases

- are diagnosed with advanced disease, which is affected by either treatment or disease progression. Stoma surgery is performed, either as an elective procedure for symptom relief, such as fistulae, or as an emergency for intestinal obstruction (see Chapter 5).

These patients who undergo surgery to alleviate problems are, in addition, confronted with changes to their normal physical appearance. Some patients may have difficulty in achieving the skills needed for stoma care management. These difficulties in skill acquisition may result from the task involved, specific circumstances or insufficient information about what to do. Physical and psychological assistance from a significant carer may be necessary; information and support to increase self-efficacy are required to enable the patients to cope socially and emotionally. Adjustment and adaptation can take considerable time, and often these patients have restricted time and/or are unable to complete this process. The speed at which nursing and medical staff facilitate this process is vital.

Receiving treatments for progression or recurrence of disease, such as radiotherapy or analgesia, can affect stomal activity. Assessment should determine the cause and whether the recurrence is temporary or permanent. Other considerations include the patient's ability to eat, drink or take medication. If bowel surgery has previously been performed, establish the level of bowel function after surgery. The presence of disease recurrence will influence treatment (see Chapter 10 for symptom management).

Diet and the stoma

Chapter 11 contains detailed information on the nutritional aspects of bowel cancer and the implications of treatment and disease state. Postoperatively nutritional needs will be supplemented intravenously, usually until bowel motility is re-established, which is identified when the bowel sounds are observed or flatus is passed. Small increased amounts of oral fluids are given and observed for tolerance, progressing to solid foods that are low in fibre, reducing peristaltic activity and the production of flatus. Dietary intake is gradually moderated to meet requirements, avoiding spicy and highly seasoned foods. The gut at this stage is unable to tolerate foods that are not easily digested. Digestive function may take several weeks to re-establish and settle down. Generally the introduction of additional foods to the diet should be spaced out; if intestinal upset does occur the 'culprit food' is readily identified and reintroduced at a later time.

Eating usually causes few problems if the guidelines have been followed. An irregular dietary pattern can cause loose and frequent bowel movements. Once the problem has been identified, appropriate treatment can usually resolve the issue, raising patient awareness on how future problems can be avoided. Individuals will have dietary preferences and cultural restrictions which may require some modification initially, and are dependent in the long term on the type of stoma and the disease state. Advice and assistance may be sought from a nutritionist, but unless indicated an experienced nurse or stoma care nurse should be able to provide guidance, based on the type of surgery performed, e.g. end-colostomy or end-ileostomy. This is often an opportune time for the nurse to review previous dietary habits and advise on foods that can aid recovery and future rehabilitation. Often as a result of a combination of physiological or psychosocial factors, dietary intake has been inappropriate to sustain need. Discussion on the benefits of adjusting certain aspects of diet to promote general health and well-being, in order to reduce future problems, should be highlighted but not forced.

The significance for someone with an ileostomy of maintaining an adequate fluid intake and electrolyte balance, because of problems resulting from the loss of the colon and its water-absorbing properties, should be stressed. Postoperatively, the daily output can be up to 1500 ml, gradually decreasing to around 350–800 ml (Black 2000), often resembling a toothpaste or porridge consistency depending on the type of dietary and fluid intake. Likewise, awareness is needed of those foods with a high fibrous content that may cause blockage of the small intestine's narrow lumen (bolus obstruction) if not adequately chewed or digested; these include pineapple, sweetcorn, rice, nuts, mushrooms, celery, vegetables and fruit skins.

A person with a colostomy can firm up a loose stool by eating foods high in fibre, typically wholemeal-, wheat- and oat-based products. Bananas, marshmallows or gelatine-derived foods are useful to thicken a loose stool for either a colostomy or an ileostomy.

Discharge preparation and ongoing needs

Increasingly the period of hospital stay is shorter as a result of political, administrative and financial pressures. Preparation for discharge is central to care, starting preoperatively with family involvement throughout all the stages of the process. Most patients, throughout their period of hospitalization, look forward to going home to a familiar social setting. After stoma surgery this denotes a major step in recovery.

Ongoing assessment and evaluation will have identified potential self-care deficits, which will not be wholly resolved until rehabilitation is complete. Communication and liaison with appropriate members of the multidisciplinary team, such as GPs, district nurses, and the statutory and voluntary services, are essential. Specialist nurses such as stoma, palliative and oncology nurses have a pivotal role, working between the boundaries of primary and secondary care, and are ideally placed to support continuity and ongoing care. Patients should be given the contact details of those support services involved in their ongoing care, including the stoma care nurse. A supply of stoma equipment is given on discharge, together with details of future requirements and how equipment is obtained. UK citizens aged over 60 (female) or 65 years (male) with a permanent stoma are exempt from prescription costs and may require an exemption form.

Table 9.4 Stoma care discharge preparation record

Hospital number

Name	Date of surgery	Type of stoma
Address	Diagnosis	
Consultant	GP	
SCN Tel. no	Community nurse	Tel. no
Other agencies involved		
Literature		

Perineal wound	Peristomal skin	
Stoma condition	Yes/No	Comments
Discharge/transfer date		
Sutures out		
Competent in stoma management/disposal		
Aware of common complications		
Prescription details/exemption form		
Appliances given		
Storage of appliances		
Radiotherapy/chemotherapy		
Voluntary organizations		
Home visit		
Other agencies		
Stoma clinic appointment		

Stoma care management record

Action	Dependent	With assistance	Supervised	Independent	Comments
1. Stoma observation and familiarization of specific appliance and clip					
2. Drainage of appliance and correctly reapplies clip					
3. Removal of soiled appliance cleansing of skin and stoma					
4. Preparation of a correctly fitting appliance					
5. Application of appliance					
6. Complete procedure, i.e. removal of used appliance, applies new appliance correctly					
7. Appropriate method of disposal discussed					
8. Written contact details given on how to obtain help and support					

The goals for discharge planning (Table 9.4) can be summarized as follows (Allison 1996, p. 268):

1. Enable people to return home
2. Effective stoma care and management
3. Facilitate reintegration into the community setting
4. Enable people to maintain, physical, psychological and social rehabilitation.

Disposal

Guidance is necessary for an acceptable method of appliance disposal. Initial assessment will have identified issues relating to the patient's environment and the provision of specific facilities for disposal of body waste. Generally, faecal waste from pouches should be emptied down the lavatory; appliances should be rinsed through and placed in a polythene bag and disposed of in household waste. Alternatives include commercially produced 'disposal units' or services provided by the local authority. These issues need to be raised before discharge.

Dealing with common stoma problems

An important part of patient and carer education is raising awareness and recognition of changes relating to the stoma and when to seek advice. Nurses are ideally placed to help patients check for actual and potential problems. Stoma appliances should provide adequate adhesion and confidence to reduce trauma and leakage. Appliances should be renewed regularly to prevent seepage and skin trauma, but not recurrently to create skin damage. Problems most frequently encountered are changes relating to the stoma, described below, and usually happen in the community within the first year after surgery.

Trauma and infection

Frequently, skin excoriation can present soon after the patient's return home and prompt action should be taken before the problem has exacerbated. Sore skin underneath an appliance can make pouch adhesion and management difficult. A leaking appliance can have a devastating effect on patient morale and psychological well-being. Assessment should include patient technique, appliance fitting and appropriateness, any underlying skin condition that had not previously been apparent, dietary intake and stoma output. Shrinkage of stoma size in the weeks after surgery is expected, and patient teaching should emphasize the importance of regular stoma measurement. Too large an aperture, exposing skin immediately surrounding the stoma, is a common cause of skin soreness. Smith et al. (2002) state that allergic dermatitis is an uncommon reason for peristomal skin conditions as a result of effective technological developments in the production of stoma products. The prevailing cause of irritant skin reactions is attributed to effluent spillage. This study indicated that about 50% of patients described an inappropriate aperture size as the cause of their skin soreness.

Skin infection usually needs topical treatment which can affect appliance adhesion. An occlusive dressing positioned over the affected area enables pouch adhesion.

Retraction

This is commonly associated with weight gain after surgery, where the stoma appears to be bounded by skin folds. Other causes include poor fixation of the bowel through the abdominal wall. According to Wade (1989), this accounted for 7.6% of problems in patients within 10 weeks of surgery. Conservative management technique includes a convex pouching method, which helps the stoma to protrude. If unsuccessful, refashioning of the stoma may be required.

Stenosis

Stenosis is a narrowing of the opening for faecal discharge and, if untreated, can cause obstruction. Effluent 'pools' around the stoma, causing leakage and skin soreness. This problem can occur months or years after surgery, usually linked to earlier complications. Short-term measures include using convex pouching systems and skin protective agents with local stoma dilatation; this is usually unsatisfactory and successful treatment requires refashioning of the stoma (Irving and Hume 1993, p. 70).

Hernia

Generally, a parastomal hernia can potentially occur anywhere along the surgical incision. Other indications include ineffective abdominal muscle control. A non-invasive technique such as the use of an abdominal support belt that accommodates the stoma is commonly advised. Surgical repair may be necessary as a long-term measure, particularly when stoma management becomes a problem.

Prolapse

The transverse colostomy is most prone to this complication, with an eventual 20% being affected (Borwell 1994, 2004). A prolapsed stoma is a startling experience for patient and carer, particularly if the distal and proximal loops are involved. In most instances, the transverse colostomy is created as a temporary measure with ultimate closure. Manual reduction may be possible. Where this is a recurring problem, patients can sometimes be taught the technique, ensuring that the appliance is *in situ* to allow the prolapsed stoma to fall correctly into position (Torrence 1997).

Conclusion

Changes in the way cancer care is organized have the potential not only to improve the outcome of treatment but also to streamline the appropriate evaluation of breakthrough cancer treatment that is anticipated from the rapidly advancing knowledge of cancer biology.

Any long- or short-term chronic illness almost immediately becomes the main focus of a person's life, involving family members having to make changes that disrupt life's usual pattern. Strong emotions may be experienced; anger is often directed at loved ones. It is difficult for most people to understand and some partners may see a slow transformation of someone they have loved into someone in whom affections have changed and with whom they can no longer live. All situations are different and some carers even thrive on the extra attention and responsibility (Anon 2002). Nurses are in an ideal position to support the needs of carers, through liaison and access to other resources and welfare agencies (see Chapter 14).

Managing colorectal cancer is complex and challenging, but, with suitable care, comprehensive patient education and psychosocial support, improvements can be made to a patient's quality of life which increases chances of survival from the disease.

Summary of key points

- Quality of care is essentially a matter of values and measurement. As the health service becomes more resource-minded, health professionals need to make sure that quality of care is their prime objective.
- Integrated care pathways provide clinicians with a systematic process to manage patient care. Further research is needed to establish their effect on patient outcomes and the impact on nursing practice.

- Nursing's contribution to society is concerned with meeting the needs of the person, the family and the community.
- Specifically focused information about treatment options, side effects and prognosis is predominantly significant, and can facilitate psychological adaptation.
- Patients requiring stoma formation have particular considerations.
- Nurses have a pivotal role in discharge preparation and ongoing care.

References

Allison M (1996) Discharge planning for the person with a stoma. In: Myers C (ed.), Stoma Care Nursing: A patient-centred approach. London: Edward Arnold.

Anon (2002) In it together. Nursing Standard 16(22): 27.

Black P (2000) Holistic Stoma Care. London: Baillière Tindall.

Borwell B (1994) Practical management of bowel stomas. Nursing Standard 8(45): 49-56.

Borwell B (1997) Psychological considerations of stoma care nursing. Nursing Standard 11(48): 49-53.

Borwell B (1999) Sexuality and stoma care. In: Taylor P (ed.), Stoma Care in the Community. London: Nursing Times Books.

Borwell B (2004) Bowel stomas: how and when they are created. In: Breckman B (ed.), Stoma Care, 2nd edn. London: Elsevier, in press.

Boyd-Carson W, Thompson MJ, Boyd K (2004) Mucocutaneous separation: clinical protocols for stoma care: 4. Nursing Standard 18(17): 41-3.

Breckman B (1998) Stoma management. In: Doyle D, Hanks GWC, MacDonald N (eds), Oxford: Oxford University Press, pp. 839-45

Buggins E (1995) Mind your language. Nursing Standard 10(1): 21-2.

Cancer Services Collaborative (2001) Bowel Cancer: The patient journey: service improvement guides. London: Department of Health: www.nelh.nhs.uk/nsf/cancer/bowel_sig/summary/figure.1htm (accessed update).

Cavanagh SJ (1991) Orem's Model in Action. London: Macmillan.

Coulter A, Entwhistle V, Gilbert D (1999) Sharing decisions with patients: is the information good enough? Journal of Advanced Nursing 318: 318-22.

Crossfield T (1989) How to formulate patient assessment. Nursing Standard 3(44): 45.

Department of Health (1997) The NHS: Modern, Dependable. London: The Stationery Office.

Department of Health (1998) A First Class Service: Quality in the new NHS. London: The Stationery Office.

Department of Health (2000a) The NHS Plan: A plan for investment, a plan for reform. London: The Stationery Office.

Department of Health (2000b) The NHS Cancer Plan. London: The Stationery Office.

Department of Health (2003) Cancer Services Collaborative: Improvement partnership. A quick guide. London: The Stationery Office.

Edwards E, Miller C (2001) Improving psychosocial assessment in oncology. Professional Nurse 16: 1223-6.

Entwhistle VA, Watt IS, Sowden AJ (1997) Information to facilitate patient involvement in decision making: some issues. Journal of Clinical Effectiveness 2(3): 69-72.

Grahn G (1996) Patient information as a necessary therapeutic intervention. European Journal of Cancer Care 5(suppl 1): 1-8.

Graydon J, Galloway S, Palmer-Wickham S (1997) Information needs of women during early treatment for breast cancer. Journal of Advanced Nursing 26: 59-67.

Guezo J (2003) Total abdominal hysterectomy: development of a patient-centred care pathway. Nursing Standard 18(3): 38-42.

Henley A, Schott J (1999) Culture, Religion and Patient Care in a Multi-Ethnic Society. London: Age Concern.

Hunter D (1995) Panacea or placebo? Health Service Journal 105: 22–4.

Irving MH, Hume O (1993) Intestinal stomas. In: Jones DJ, Irving MH (eds), ABC of Colorectal Diseases. London: BMJ Publishing Group, pp. 68–70.

Isaksen AS, Thuen F, Hanestad B (2003) Patients with cancer and their close relatives. Cancer Nursing 26(1): 68–74.

Kelly M (1992) Self, identity and radical surgery. Sociology of Health and Illness 14: 390–415.

Ley P (1995) Communicating with Patients. London: Chapman & Hall.

McCahon S (1999) Faecal stomas. In: Porritt T, Daniel N (eds), Essential Coloproctology for Nurses. London: Whurr Publishers.

Mckenzie FD, Ingram VA (2001) Dansac Invent convex in the management of flush ileostomy. British Journal of Nursing 10: 1005–9.

Mills ME, Sullivan K (1999) The importance of information giving for patients newly diagnosed with cancer: a review of the literature. Journal of Clinical Nursing 8: 631–42.

National Cancer Alliance (1996) Patient Centred Services? What patients say. Oxford: National Cancer Alliance.

National Cancer Guidance Steering Group (2004) Improving Outcomes in Colorectal Cancer Update Manual. London: NICE.

National Institute for Clinical Excellence (2003) Factsheet: General information about clinical guidelines. London: NICE.

Nursing and Midwifery Council (2002) Code of Professional Conduct. London: NMC.

Orem DE (1991) Nursing Concepts of Practice, 4th edn. New York: McGraw-Hill.

Royal College of Nursing (2002) Caring for people with colorectal problems. Report of the RCN/Coloplast Competencies Project. London: RCN.

Royal College of Radiologists (2003) When cancer runs in the family: news review. *i* can Autumn (7): 4 (www.goingfora.com, www.ican4u.com).

Smith AJ, Lyon C, Hart CA (2002) Multidisciplinary care of skin problems in stoma patients. Urostomy Association Journal 65: 35–8.

Soloman MJ, Pager CK, Findlay M et al. (2003) What do patients want? Patient preferences and surrogate decision making in the treatment of colorectal cancer. Diseases of the Colon and Rectum 46: 1351–7.

Sprangers M, Taal BG, Aaronson NK et al. (1995) Quality of life in colorectal cancer: stoma v no stoma patients. Diseases of the Colon and Rectum 38: 361–9.

Torrence C (1997) Surgical Nursing, 12th edn. London: Baillière Tindall.

Wade B (1989) A Stoma is for Life. Harrow: Scutari Press.

Useful reading

Black P (2000) Holistic Stoma Care. London: Baillière Tindall.

National Institute for Clinical Excellence (2004) Improving Supportive and Palliative Care for Adults with Cancer. London: NICE.

Penson J, Fisher RA (2002) Palliative Care for People with Cancer, 3rd edn. London: Arnold.

Web address

National Pathways Association available at: www.the-npa.org.uk

Chapter 10

Continuity and community care

Catherine Hughes

Within the field of cancer care there is increasing emphasis on the role of the primary care team in ensuring the continuity of care and meeting the needs of patients and carers (Expert Advisory Group on Cancer 1995). Patients with a diagnosis of cancer may spend only short periods of time in hospital, but the majority of their lives will be spent at home (Department of Health or DoH 2000). This indicates the importance of the primary health-care team in taking the lead in the continuing care of patients with a cancer diagnosis. For many patients with a diagnosis of cancer, their physical, emotional, spiritual, social and financial stability may be considerably challenged. The psychological and physical consequences of a cancer diagnosis can threaten a person's sense of well-being and quality of life (McDonald 2001). Some people with a diagnosis of bowel cancer can expect a relatively long and worthwhile remission or cure, whereas the future prognosis for those patients with advanced disease is likely to be poor; about 50% of patients presenting with a colorectal adenocarcinoma will die from metastatic disease (Young and Rea 2001).

Patients diagnosed with bowel cancer move through a number of health-care settings during the course of their illness, encountering many health professionals. A successful transition through these settings depends on the collaborative efforts of the health-care providers. Although the primary care team are involved with health promotion, prevention and diagnosis (see Chapter 2), the aim of this chapter is to highlight the continuity and community needs of these patients after surgery/treatment and throughout the cancer experience. It gives an overview of how continuity of care can be achieved and the resources available to improve both the physical and the psychosocial well-being of patients and carers, with emphasis on patients with advanced disease. It also highlights the palliative and terminal care needs of this client group, including bereavement considerations.

Communication and team working

Ongoing communication and collaboration are the key to continuity of care. The document *Guidance on Supportive and Palliative Care* (National Institute for Clinical Excellence or NICE 2004) identifies the communication essential to deliver effective supportive and palliative care services. *The Calman–Hine Report* (Expert Advisory Group on Cancer 1995) states the importance of communication between primary care and specialist services. The report recognized that primary care not only provides psychological and emotional support but also acts as a formal link between patients and cancer services. McCann (1998) makes the point that the report emphasizes that communication should be appropriate in both time and content. General practitioners and district nurses are key carers for the patient and it is important that they are involved in the care of individuals from the day of diagnosis. It is recommended that discharge information should reach the relevant members of the primary health-care team on the day of discharge (Expert Advisory Group on Cancer 1995). Communication with the nursing teams from hospital to community is often made by hospital community liaison nurses, by fax or telephone, on the day of discharge. To ensure all appropriate community care facilities are assembled, it would be appropriate for hospital personnel to liaise with the community team once the discharge date has been decided. It is essential for relevant information to be given; this should include the patient's diagnosis and understanding of the disease, management plan, drugs prescribed and other agencies involved. GPs are often notified of discharge via a discharge summary. This is either posted or given to the patient to deliver and can often take time to reach the relevant physician. If GP involvement is required, the use of fax or telephone is important (McCann 1998). It must be emphasized that communication is a two-way process and that it is essential for the primary care team to communicate effectively and collaborate with hospital staff before admission. The participation of patients and carers in the decision-making process when planning discharge is essential; likewise, when arrangements are made this should be effectively communicated.

According to Higginson (1999), clients, families and health professionals agree that there is a need for regular communication between all parties. This ensures the smooth transition between services, facilitates continuity of care, avoids service duplication, improves the quality of care and provides patient control. Communication between primary and secondary care is essential throughout the patient's cancer journey. In some areas of the country, patient-held records are being used. These records provide information about the updated treatment plan for individual patients and can be viewed by health professionals and others involved in their care. They have been acknowledged as a useful information and communication tool for patients, carers and health professionals (McCann 1998, Johnson 2002). The introduction of electronic communication systems between hospitals and primary care trusts should bring improvements in the two-way communication process, because they provide a speedy, cost-saving and effective form of transmission (Closs 1997).

A multiprofessional team-working approach is essential to ensure continuity and coordination of care among all those involved in meeting the needs of patients with cancer. Henneman et al. (1995) state that a lack of collaboration can lead to a fragmentation of patient care, patient dissatisfaction, poor outcomes and job dissatisfaction for health professionals. The Gold Standard Framework (GSF) is a structure to improve the organization and quality of palliative care services for patients who are at home in the last years of their life; targeted specifically at primary health-care teams, and currently being introduced across the UK, it is an ongoing development (Macmillan Cancer Relief 2003). One of the aims of the GSF is to implement proactive planning for out-of-hours care; this has the potential to prevent unnecessary emergency admissions and facilitates patient choice of place of care or death. Team work, job satisfaction, communication and co-working with specialists and hospital teams will also be improved. Although the GSF is aimed specifically at cancer patients in their last 6–12 months of life, in the future it could be extended to cancer patients from the point of diagnosis (Macmillan Cancer Relief 2003).

One way to ensure continuity of care is to identify a key worker to act as a coordinator for the patient, family, health-care professionals and other agencies involved. The health-care professional who has maximum patient contact is normally the most suitable; this member could be from either the secondary or the primary care team. The key worker may change to reflect a patient's changing needs.

A patient with bowel cancer may need supportive care from different health professionals and other agencies, depending on the stage of the disease, surgical intervention, treatment, and the physical and psychosocial needs of the patient and carers. Even those discharged from hospital, considered to be of low dependency, could benefit from community team involvement. A study undertaken by Van Hartfeveld et al. (1997) looked at 337 patients with cancer, where a district nurse referral would not usually be made. Every patient was offered a visit from the community nursing team. The results of the study identified that 93% of patients experienced some physical or psychosocial problems that had not been identified in hospital. Both patients and nurses found the visit beneficial. Home visits allow the nurse to view the patient in a holistic way and assess for actual or potential problems; however, there may be some patients and carers who decline support from community services.

Bowel cancer is more prevalent among older people and the prevalence increases with age. The incidence of colorectal cancer is more common in people aged over 60 years (Cancer Research UK 2003). This indicates that many patients and carers may have other health-related physical and psychosocial needs, unrelated to their cancer. Community and continuity of care aim to ensure that patients have effective and appropriate support to promote self-care and independence to maintain quality of life, enabling them to remain at home if they desire. Establishing the needs of patients and carers holistically assists in the identification of any necessary resources to ensure that continuity of care is achieved. NICE (2004) defines service models, which recommend the support and care that cancer patients and their families want/need to enable them to cope with cancer and treatment at all the stages of illness.

General practitioners

On average a GP will only see one new case of bowel cancer a year (Hobbs 2001). Patients will have probably known the GP for some considerable time and may identify him or her as a main source of information, support and ongoing care. The most important aspect of bowel cancer is early detection and referral, together with palliation of symptoms when they arise.

The hospital surgeon or oncologist usually undertakes the surveillance of patients after a diagnosis of bowel cancer. Research has identified that there is no reliable evidence on the value of follow-up in the detection of recurrence and progression of colorectal cancer after primary treatment (NHS Executive 1997). The NHS Executive report *Improving Outcomes in Colorectal Cancer* (1997) recommends that GPs and patients be aware of the signs and symptoms that might indicate recurrence, and should any problems occur there should be referral to the colorectal MDT by the specified pathway for prompt review (National Cancer Guidance Steering Group or NCGSG 2004). This indicates that colorectal cancer surveillance could be undertaken within primary care, given appropriate training and communication between primary and secondary care.

Genetics

Advances in genetic science have an impact on the primary care team. As a result of media coverage, people seek advice because they are anxious about the increased risk of developing cancer when there is a family history of the disease. The importance of cancer genetics has been recognized by the government in *The NHS Cancer Plan* (DoH 2000) which recommends improvements to these services. *The Calman–Hine Report* (Expert

Advisory Group on Cancer 1995) recognized primary care as the principal focus for clinical genetics. The report also identified the need for education, technological developments and referral guidelines to assist this process. The primary care team needs to develop their roles to include genetic screening, basic family history advice and risk assessment, referral and ongoing support to those with a genetic condition.

District nurses

Community nurses usually work within small teams alongside other members of the primary care team. The district nurse is the predominant carer for patients in their home environment, and ideally placed to embrace collaboration between other health and social agency providers. In contrast with the GP, studies indicate that a district nurse is the professional most aware of patient and carer needs (Grande et al. 1996). Initial and ongoing assessments allow district nurses to identify the actual or potential needs of the patient and carer. Changes within the role have moved away from the provision of personal social care to that of patient assessor, aiming to facilitate independence, health and well-being. Patients with bowel cancer often have complex needs and require intervention from specialist services and other agencies. To enable the delivery of appropriate and effective care nurses need to be knowledgeable about the availability of community and hospital resources. For community nurses to provide effective palliative and supportive care, it is essential that education is provided to increase their knowledge and awareness. Education from specialist palliative care providers has been in evidence through network funding supported by the government, identified by *The NHS Cancer Plan* (DoH 2000).

Colorectal clinical nurse specialists

The numbers of colorectal nurse specialists (CNSs) employed in the UK have increased since the publication of *Improving Outcomes in Colorectal Cancer* (NHS Executive, 1997). This trend will continue because the key recommendations from the revised edition (NCGSG 2004) state that **all** patients diagnosed with colorectal cancer should have access to a named nurse with specialist knowledge of cancer at all stages of the pathway, to provide counselling and continuity of care. After diagnosis the CNS is often the first point of contact for patients and their relatives. McCreaddie (2001) identified that the nature of a clinical nurse specialist's role allows time to tailor advice and support to an individual's needs. The CNS is a central feature of the team, based on her or his in-depth knowledge of colorectal cancer and its management, and is in an ideal position to ensure coordination, collaboration and ongoing support (NCGSG 2004). The CNS is also a first point of contact for those 'disease-free' patients who may have concerns in the future.

Stoma nurse specialist

Formation of a permanent or temporary stoma may be necessary for some patients diagnosed with bowel cancer (see Chapter 5). These patients have to cope not only with bowel cancer but also with the physical and psychological impact of a stoma. The psychological effect may range from adjustment to a changed body image to anxiety and depression (White 1998). In addition, studies suggest that the incidence of psychosocial problems is increased compared with non-stoma patients (Sprangers et al. 1995). The NHS Executive (1997) recommends that patients who may require a stoma should have involvement from a specialist nurse, to offer patients and their carers support and education from the preoperative phase, through to rehabilitation (see Chapter 9). Most stoma care nurses (SCNs) work within the community and hospital settings. Working in this manner allows the SCN to act as a coordinator of care from hospital to home. Effective communication between health professionals and other primary care agencies will ensure that patients receive the support and care required (Taylor 1999). After discharge care is ongoing, with outpatient appointments and planned home visits. Pringle and Swan (2001) identified that home visits 7 days after discharge are beneficial because patients often experience stomal complications, and physical and psychological symptoms; subsequent visits are advised at 6 months and 1 year after surgery.

Community nurses have a valuable role to play in the rehabilitation of these patients. It is therefore essential that they have an understanding of stoma care and are able to recognize physical, psychological and social problems and have contact details of the SCN for specialist advice and support.

Community cancer nurse specialists and cancer centres

Some patients with a diagnosis of bowel cancer will require adjuvant, neoadjuvant or palliative chemotherapy or radiotherapy (see Chapters 6 and 7). With advances in technology, treatment and improved venous access devices, patients may have the option of receiving chemotherapy at home or in an outpatient setting. Patients with bowel cancer fall into this category either in the form of ambulatory chemotherapy such as continuous infusion of 5-fluorouracil (5FU) and oral capecitabine. The main advantages of having chemotherapy at home include convenience, not having to travel, reduced anxiety and less disruption to normal activities (Rischin et al. 2000).

It is essential that patients and carers of those eligible for possible home chemotherapy are carefully selected and receive specialist education relating to the care of the central venous access device and infusion pumps, and the potential side effects of treatment (Dougherty 1998). This will have an impact on the community team and requires close collaboration. Problems associated with community-based continuous ambulatory chemotherapy are mostly manageable with efficient support from district nurses and the GP (Dougherty 1998). Pre-discharge preparation and communication with the community team are essential to maintain continuity. There is little evidence for identifying how this can best be achieved. Supplying a copy of the information given to the patient, and advice about how to manage side effects and care of the central venous access, would assist in ensuring continuity of care. It is also recommended that the primary care team and patients have 24-hour access to information and advice from oncology-trained staff (NHS Executive 1997).

Community-based cancer nurse specialists have been employed in some areas of the UK. These nurses are designated to individual practices and provide information and support for cancer patients (Dawson 1999, Wood 1999, Glover 2000). Based on a satisfactory pilot study in Dorset (Dawson 1999), five cancer nurse specialists were employed by Poole Primary Care Trust. Aiming to bridge the gap between primary and secondary care, strong links have been established between the community team and the local cancer centre. Their duties appertaining to bowel cancer include changing of continuous infusional pumps, monitoring for any treatment side effects, and providing patient information and psychological support. Assistance is also given in the management of central venous access devices, emphasizing the need for patient education in self-care or community nursing teams in the management of the devices used, and about primary information and seamless care. Formal evaluation of the service has not yet been undertaken.

Patients with a rectal tumour who receive adjuvant or neoadjuvant radiotherapy may experience side effects (see Chapter 7). Treatment is usually given on an outpatient basis for side effects that persist after treatment; these patients will need ongoing support from the community team. It is essential that the team are familiar with current information and research about potential side effects and their management. Community staff should contact the radiotherapy department or members of the oncology team if they need advice and support.

A patient considered 'disease free' may need minimal input from the primary care team once normal activities are resumed.

Palliative/supportive care

Palliative care concerns the relief of physical and psychological distress. It is best defined by the World Health Organization (WHO 1990, p. 11):

> Palliative care is the active total care of patients whose disease is not responsive to curative treatment. Control of pain, and other symptoms including psychological, social and spiritual problems is paramount. The goal of palliative care is the achievement of the best quality of life for patients and their families. Many aspects of palliative care are also applicable earlier in the course of the illness in conjunction with other treatments.

Supportive care is, however, described by the National Council for Hospices and Specialist Palliative Care Services (NCHSPCS 2002) as:

> ... that which helps the patient and their family to cope with cancer and treatment of it from pre-diagnosis, through the process of diagnosis and treatment, to cure, continuing illness or death and into bereavement. It helps the patient to maximise the benefits of treatment and to live as well as possible with the effects of the disease. It is given equal priority alongside diagnosis and treatment.

Patients with advanced bowel cancer need frequent monitoring of physical and psychosocial symptoms and a multiprofessional approach is essential. GPs and other primary care team members are central to the delivery of community palliative care services; however, palliative care represents a small proportion of an individual GP's caseload, and consequently it is unrealistic to expect him or her to have the expert skills and knowledge needed (Barclay 1997). Access to palliative care services is an important source of support for the primary care team.

Palliative care teams

The National Institute for Clinical Excellence recognize that patients with advanced disease often suffer from a range of complex problems that may require specialist palliative care services (NICE 2004). Supportive care should involve local palliative care services both in the community and in the hospital. Contact with the palliative team should ideally be made at the time of diagnosis in a patient with advanced disease, not when a crisis occurs (Young and Rea 2001).

Services provided by palliative teams are varied and each should include a palliative care nurse and consultant in palliative care (NHS Executive 1997). These teams usually have access to other services, which may include inpatient (hospice) and day-care facilities. There is a range of other services and resources to be accessed by patients and carers that are linked to the palliative care team, such as counselling, social workers, dietitians, physiotherapy, occupational therapy, alternative therapies, chaplaincy, clinical psychologists and bereavement services.

The community specialist palliative care nurse provides advice, support and education to primary care teams, other workers in primary care, patients and carers. Equipped with specialist knowledge and expertise, they are able to offer emotional and practical support for patients and carers; for the health professional they are a valuable resource on symptom control and management. These nurses are frequently linked with the community and hospices. This provides an easily accessible patient referral route between GPs and palliative care consultants. In situations where complex symptom management cannot be supported at home or when respite care is required, admission arrangements to the hospital, hospice or palliative care unit can be explored.

Disease recurrence in those patients with advanced bowel cancer is most commonly linked with liver or peritoneal metastases, or both; these can sometimes metastasize to the lungs; cerebral or bone metastases are rare (Taylor et al. 2002). These patients may have symptoms associated with disease progression, which may include pain, nausea and vomiting, loss of appetite, ascites, constipation, jaundice, breathing difficulties and fatigue. Those patients with pelvic recurrence may also have symptoms such as tenesmus and necrotic tumour protruding through the peritoneum, which can cause great distress. Psychosocial indicators can include fear, anxiety, anger, stress and guilt. Specialist palliative care assessment may be required to reduce or eliminate symptoms. Such procedures can be simplified for patients if a baseline assessment was undertaken at an earlier stage of the disease. In the interim patients may be discharged home.

Unfortunately there are times when admission to a hospital or hospice is required as a result of a lack of appropriate community services. Dependent on locally available resources, there are other health professionals and agencies that can provide this support at home.

Social Services

Following the NHS and Community Care Act recommendations (DoH 1990), the responsibility for patients with personal care needs has moved from the district nursing team to Social Services (see Chapter 14). There may come a point when the patient is unable to undertake normal activities of daily living, or management exceeds the limitations of the carer, requiring support from Social Services. District nurses undertaking continual assessment of individual patient's and carer's needs may refer on to Social Services to prevent hospital admission enabling them to remain at home. Assessment of individual need by a home care manager will establish and initiate the relevant support. Service costs are dependent on a patient's financial status. Services available include assistance with personal care, shopping, housekeeping and making meals. Social Services can also arrange 'meals on wheels' and frozen packaged meals. Another facility determined by individual need is the installation of an emergency 24-hour alarm system.

Occupational therapist/physiotherapist

Referrals from the district nursing service to an occupational therapist or physiotherapist may be necessary when practical equipment, mobility aids or home modifications are required to allow the patient to remain at home. The community occupational team or physiotherapist, following an assessment of the home and a patient's physical ability, would provide appropriate equipment, e.g. commode, wheelchair, mechanical hoist, raised toilet seat or bathing aids. Each individual oncology patient should be given the opportunity to achieve his or her optimal level of independence through access to a state-registered occupational therapist who can provide assessment and treatment of physical, social, cognitive and environmental difficulties in the community (Cranfield and McMillan 1998). Some areas of the country have access to rapid response community rehabilitation teams. NICE (2004) recommend that equipment required by a patient nearing the end of life should be made available within 24 hours of the request being made.

Respite care

Carers take on a lot of responsibility when caring for a person with life-threatening illness. Payne et al. (1999) identified that there is considerable physical, psychological, social and financial challenge in being a carer for someone nearing the end of life. One approach to overcome these and associated problems is to offer respite care. This can be given by using appropriate physical and practical help available through services previously discussed, and hospice at home schemes, inpatient care or day care, or utilization of voluntary sector resources.

Palliative care units or hospices can ideally provide short-term respite admission to assist the carer; however, as a result of a deficiency in inpatient facilities this is frequently unachievable, and nursing homes are often used as an alternative. Hospice day-care facilities expanded rapidly in the UK between 1980 and 1990, increasing from 11 to 251 day units (Higginson et al. 2000). This service provides patients with a 'day out' and carers with a day of respite. Amenities are variable and include rehabilitation facilities, creative and therapeutic activities, emotional support, assessment, symptom management, social interaction, access to services such as alternative therapies, counsellor, dietitian, physiotherapist and occupational therapist.

In addition there are national voluntary organizations, such as Marie Curie Cancer Care, which are able to provide a 24-hour, 'hands-on', palliative nursing service. Unfortunately, this is a limited resource because of staff availability and restricted funding. A member of the primary care team, mainly the district nurse, usually initiates referral. Marie Curie nurses are not palliative care specialists but nurses with advanced general and palliative care skills. District nurse assessment will identify the level of expertise required because not all these nurses hold a qualification governed by the Nursing and Midwifery Council (NMC 2002). The Marie Curie nurse offers physical care, monitors symptom management, and gives medication (where appropriate) and emotional support. Other voluntary schemes depend on local provision (see Chapter 14).

Financial concerns can be an extra stressor for some people with the additional costs incurred by extra service provision. Historically, the social worker usually dealt with assessment of financial remuneration; currently this can be initiated by any health professional. People with bowel cancer may be entitled to benefits such as Disability Living Allowance (DLA) for those aged under 65 years, or Attendance Allowance (AA) for those over 65. If the prognosis is thought to be less than 6 months, special rules apply; the GP should include a DS1500 with each application form to ensure that financial assistance is provided as quickly as possible. The Citizens Advice Bureau and social workers are a good resource for advice about other benefit entitlements (see Chapter 14).

Terminal care

The death of a terminally ill patient can often be anticipated; patients and carers need the opportunity to express any fears or anxieties. Signs often associated in cancer patients with the dying phase of disease are immobility, decrease in consciousness and when the intake of oral fluids or medication is no longer possible (Ellershaw and Ward 2003). An explanation of this progressive loss of consciousness and management of symptoms may relieve some of the anxiety experienced by the patient and carer.

Research shows that most people, when given the choice, would prefer to die at home. Statistics suggest that 60% of cancer patients in the UK would favour this option (Office for National Statistics 2001); however, in 1999 this was achieved in only 24% of patients (Office for National Statistics 2002). In the UK most patients with bowel cancer die at home (Hobbs 2001).

If a patient wishes to stay at home, it is essential that appropriate services and resources are instigated, as discussed earlier. A study by Higginson and Wilkinson (2002) identified that 90% of patients who received care from a Marie Curie nurse died at home. This indicates that an increase in resources has the potential to allow more patients to fulfil their final choice. It is essential to have an emergency supply of drugs in the home to alleviate symptoms that could occur and to allay any fears or distress caused by uncontrolled symptoms.

Sometimes dying at home is not possible for practical reasons, such as uncontrolled symptoms, lack of resources and support to ensure appropriate care to patients and carers, or a change of preference by either patient or carer on the place to die. Storey et al. (2003) identified those factors that prevent patients from dying at home; this included consistency of resources across the community served, demographic factors, the skills and knowledge of all involved in caring, carer exhaustion and regular evaluation of intended care outcomes. *The NHS Cancer Plan* (DoH 2000) acknowledged the inadequacy in some areas of palliative care; areas highlighted included poor coordination, inconsistent out-of-hours service or lack of 24-hour access to care, and insufficient training for the primary care teams. Currently the government aims to expand specialist palliative care services, and to provide additional training and support in the general principles and practice of palliative care for the primary care team. This demonstration of commitment to palliative care by the government does not resolve the problem of insufficient resources. The GSF (Macmillan Cancer Relief 2003) mentioned earlier provides a useful tool to improve these services; it may also allow more patients to remain at home. Equally significant are improvements to communication, team working and continuity of care, developing further symptom management strategies, and increasing patient, carer and staff support. The aim is to improve advanced planning opportunities to ensure that the appropriate resources are available, so avoiding crisis in care.

Bereavement

The death of a relative or someone close to you is one of the most stressful and disturbing life events that there is. Bereavement support has become an essential aspect of palliative care (Payne 2001), acknowledging that bereavement visits are recommended. The most appropriate health professional to undertake the initial visit would be the person most frequently involved in a patient's care immediately before death. These visits allow the bereaved person(s) to share emotions and allow professionals to assist by offering help, support and information. This also provides an opportunity to assess the needs of the bereaved and identify whether extra support is required to help them work through the complex and individual stages of grief. Palliative care services often provide bereavement assisted by the use of specially trained counsellors and volunteers, acting as a accessible resource if required. Voluntary organizations such as Cruse are a further contact for bereaved individuals.

Conclusion

This chapter has identified that primary care plays a significant role in caring for patients with cancer. The patient with a diagnosis of bowel cancer and the carers will encounter numerous health professionals and personnel from other agencies (Figure 10.1). It is necessary to ensure that patients, carers and health-care professionals have access to experts who have specialist skills and knowledge to promote best practice.

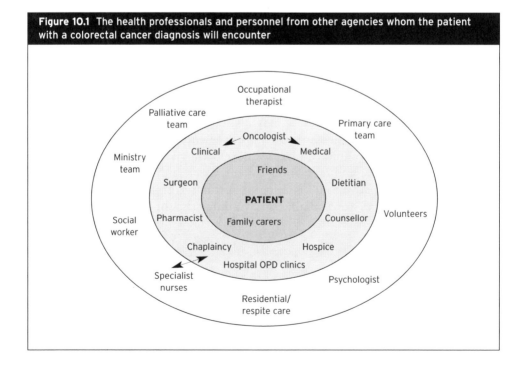

Figure 10.1 The health professionals and personnel from other agencies whom the patient with a colorectal cancer diagnosis will encounter

Summary of key points

To ensure continuity of care the following are essential:

- Communication
- Collaboration
- Coordination
- Availability of appropriate resources
- Education for primary health-care professionals in cancer care, palliative care and genetics
- Addressing physical, psychological, social and spiritual needs of the patients and families.

References

Barclay S (1997) Palliative care in the community: the role of the primary health care team. European Journal of Palliative Care 6(1): 46-7.

Black P (2000) Practical stoma care. Nursing Standard 14(41): 47-53.

Cancer Research UK (2003) Bowel cancer factsheet: www.cancerresearchuk.org/statistics.

Closs SJ (1997) Discharge communication between hospital and community health care staff: a selective review. Health and Social Care in the Community 5: 181-97.

Cranfield S, McMillan I (1998) Pathways in Cancer Care: Colorectal cancer care pathway. London: Chapman & Hall.

Dawson T (1999) A cancer nurse in the primary care setting. European Journal of Oncology Nursing 3: 251-2.

Department of Health (1990) NHS and Community Care Act. London: HMSO

Department of Health (2000) The NHS Cancer Plan. London: HMSO.

Dougherty L (1998) Establishing ambulatory chemotherapy at home. Professional Nurse 13: 356-8.

Ellershaw J, Ward C (2003) Care of the dying patient: the last hours or days of life. British Medical Journal 326: 30-4.

Expert Advisory Group on Cancer (1995) The Calman-Hine Report: A policy framework for commissioning cancer services. London: The Stationery Office.

Glover E (2000) Cancer nursing in the community. Primary Health Care 10(6): 22-4.

Grande GE, Todd J, Barclay SG et al. (1996) What terminally ill patients value in the support provided by GPs, district and Macmillan nurses. International Journal of Palliative Nursing 2: 138-43.

Henneman EA, Lee JL, Cohen JI (1995) Collaboration: a concept analysis. Journal of Advanced Nursing 21(1): 103-9.

Higginson I (1999) Palliative care services in the community: what family doctors want? Journal of Palliative Care 15(2): 21-5.

Higginson I, Wilkinson S (2002) Marie Curie nurses: enabling patients with cancer to die at home. British Journal of Community Nursing 7: 240-4.

Higginson I, Hearn J, Myers K et al. (2000) Palliative day care: what do services do? Palliative Medicine 14: 227-8.

Hobbs R (2001) The role of primary care In: Kerr DJ, Young AM, Hobbs R (eds), ABC of Colorectal Cancer. London: BMJ Books.

Johnson S (2002) A patient-held record for cancer patients from diagnosis onwards. International Journal of Palliative Nursing 8: 182-9.

McCann C (1998) Communication in cancer care: introducing patient held records. Journal of Palliative Care 15: 222-9.

McCreaddie M (2001) The role of the clinical nurse specialist. Nursing Standard 19(10): 33-8.

McDonald BH (2001) Quality of life in cancer care: patients' experiences and nurses' contribution. European Journal of Oncology Nursing 5: 32-41.

Macmillan Cancer Relief (2003) Gold Standard Framework: a programme for community palliative care. London: Macmillan Cancer Relief.

National Cancer Guidance Steering Group (2004) Improving Outcomes in Colorectal Cancer. Revised manual. London: Department of Health.

National Council for Hospices and Specialist Palliative Care Services (2002) Definitions of Supportive and Palliative Care. A consultation paper. London: NCHSPCS.

NHS Executive (1997) Improving Outcomes in Colorectal Cancer. The manual. London: Department of Health.

National Institute for Clinical Excellence (2004) Guidance on Supportive and Palliative Care; available from www.nhs.org.uk.

Nursing and Midwifery Council (2002) Code of Professional Conduct. London: NMC

Office for National Statistics (2001) Births and Deaths: Summary data. London: ONS.

Office for National Statistics (2002) Births and Deaths: Summary data. London: ONS.

Payne S (2001) Bereavement support: something for everyone? International Journal of Palliative Nursing 7: 108.

Payne S, Smith P, Dean S (1999) Identifying the concerns of informal carers in palliative care. Palliative Medicine 13: 37-44.

Pringle W, Swan E (2001) Continuing care after discharge from hospital for stoma patients. British Journal of Nursing 10: 1275-88.

Rischin D, White MA, Matthews JP et al. (2000) A randomised cross over trial of chemotherapy in the home: patient preference and cost analysis. Medical Journal of Australia 173: 125-7.

Sprangers M, Taal B, Aaronason N et al. (1995) Quality of life in colorectal cancer: stoma vs non-stoma patients. Diseases of the Colon and Rectum 38: 361-9.

Storey L, Pemberton C, Howard A (2003) Place of death: Hobson's choice or patient choice? Cancer Nursing Practice 2(4): 33-8.

Taylor I, Garcia-Aguilar J, Goldberg SM (2002) Colorectal Cancer Fast Facts, 2nd edn. Oxford: Health Press.

Taylor P (1999) Stoma Care in the Community. London: Nursing Times Books.

Van Hartfeveld JTM, Mistean PJML, Dukkers Van Emden D (1997) Home visits by community nurses for patients after discharge from hospital: An evaluation study of the community visits. Cancer Nursing 20: 105-14.

White C (1998) Psychological management of stoma related concerns. Nursing Standard 12(36): 35-6.

Wood C (1999) Cancer care in the community. Primary Health Care 9(7): 13-15.

World Health Organization (1990) Cancer Pain Relief and Palliative Care. Technical report series 804. Geneva: WHO.

Young AM, Rea D (2001) Treatment of advanced disease In: Kerr DJ, Young A M, Hobbs RFD (eds), ABC of Colorectal Cancer. London: BMJ Books.

Useful reading

Charlton R (2002) Primary Palliative Care: Dying, death and bereavement in the community. Oxon: Radcliffe Medical Press.

Hodgson SV, Maher ER (1999) A Practical Guide to Human Cancer Genetics, 2nd edn. Cambridge: Cambridge University, Press.

Thomas K (2003) Caring for the Dying at Home. Oxon: Radcliffe Medical Press.

Twycross R, Wilcock A (2002) Symptom Management in Advanced Cancer, 3rd edn. Oxon: Radcliffe Medical Press.

Chapter 11

Nutrition and bowel cancer

Emily Walters

Principles of nutrition in the cancer patient

Nutrition and the development of bowel cancer
(*see also* Chapter 1)

The relationship between diet and the development of bowel/colorectal cancer is complex. However, it is now commonly accepted that certain dietary factors are strongly implicated in the development of or the protection from the disease (World Cancer Research Fund or WCRF 1997). An estimated 90% of colorectal cancers in the USA could probably be avoided through dietary changes (Doll 1981). Obesity, particularly in men, may increase the risk of developing colorectal cancer, whereas increased physical activity is thought to be preventive. As one might predict diets high in refined carbohydrate, particularly sucrose, and fat are positively associated with development of the disease.

Epidemiological studies have shown a strong association between faecal bile acid concentration and colorectal cancer risk (Nagengast et al. 1995). Dietary fat enhances cholesterol and bile acid synthesis in the liver, thereby increasing colonic lumen sterols. Anaerobic colonic bacteria convert these sterols into cholesterol metabolites and secondary bile acids, importantly faecal bile acids. Faecal bile acids are thought to damage the colonic mucosa and increase epithelial proliferation, thereby increasing the risk of developing adenomas, the precursors to adenocarcinoma. A lower total dietary fat intake would therefore help reduce the production of faecal bile acids and the risk of colorectal malignancy.

It has been suggested that a high intake of refined carbohydrate can increase colorectal cancer risk through increased insulin resistance and hyperinsulinaemia. Obesity can also increase insulin resistance and is associated with the development of type 2 diabetes. A large epidemiological study (over 1 million participants) in the USA investigated the link between diabetes and colorectal cancer risks (Will et al. 1998). After adjustment for other colorectal cancer risk factors, the study found that men with diabetes had a 30% increased risk (significant), whereas women with diabetes had a 16% increased risk of developing colorectal cancer. However, mortality from the disease was not significantly different in those with and those without diabetes.

High intakes of alcohol and red or processed meat may also affect the development of colorectal cancer. Alcohol consumption is known to adversely affect the metabolism of folate adversely and folate deficiency is associated with increased colorectal cancer risk (Giovannucci et al. 1993). It is thought that high intakes of red or processed meat increase colonic exposure to carcinogenic agents such as N-nitroso compounds formed in the gut or heterocyclic amines formed in meat during cooking. However, it is worth noting that a comparison of five prospective studies comparing death rates in vegetarians and non-vegetarians found no significant difference in mortality from colorectal cancer (Key et al. 1999).

Dietary factors are also thought to have a protective effect against the development of colorectal malignancy. There is strong evidence to support the protective effect of a high vegetable consumption and it is commonly accepted that diets high in fibre or non-starch polysaccharides are beneficial (WCRF 1997). A high-fibre diet increases gut transit time, thereby reducing colonic mucosa exposure to dietary carcinogenic elements. The specific beneficial elements of high-fibre foods and the mechanisms by which they protect may relate to the way fibre components are used in the colon and the antioxidant properties that many high-fibre foods contain. Commonly found antioxidants known to have anti-cancer properties include micronutrients such as vitamins A, C and E, and phytochemicals such as lycopene, bioflavinoids and lutein. These are readily found in fruit and vegetables and support the advice to consume plenty of fruit and vegetables.

Colonic fermentation of soluble fibre and other dietary substrates is thought to be important in reducing colorectal cancer risk (Van Munster and Nagengast 1993). Up to 10% of starch is not digested or absorbed in the small intestine, and is therefore 'resistant' and acts as a fermentable substrate in the colon. Anaerobic fermentation of resistant starch and soluble fibre in the colon produces short-chain fatty acids (SCFAs) and promotes the production of beneficial colonic bacteria such as lactobacilli and bifidobacteria. SCFAs also create a more acidic environment in the colonic lumen by inhibiting enzymatic formation of secondary bile acids. As previously discussed, these secondary bile acids can damage the colonic mucosa, increase cell proliferation and increase the risk of developing a malignancy.

The advice for reducing colorectal cancer risks is therefore the same health promotion message as for many diseases: increased activity, maintenance of a healthy weight and consumption of a diet low in total fat and high in fibre, including at least five portions of fruit and vegetables each day (WCRF 1997).

Nutritional impact of bowel cancer

Malnutrition in cancer patients is a well-recognized problem, with studies highlighting it since the 1930s. The incidence of cachexia in cancer patients varies significantly depending on tumour site, with anorexia reported in up to 40% of patients and 80% of those with advanced disease (Wilcox et al. 1984). Many cancer patients report nutritional problems before treatment, with up to 75% of cancer patients reporting weight loss before surgery and around 50% before starting chemotherapy or radiotherapy. A retrospective study of colorectal cancer patients about to start chemotherapy found that 28% had lost 5% or more of their total body weight in the preceding 6 months. Of concern, survival was worse for those with weight loss (DeWys et al. 1980).

The cause of malnutrition in cancer patients is multifactorial and can relate to the physiological effect of the tumour, including physical obstruction, altered metabolism, iatrogenic effects of treatment and the psychological impact of diagnosis. The impact of nutritional status is far reaching, affecting both morbidity and mortality, and can affect wound healing, susceptibility to infection, recovery from surgery, length of hospital stay, response to treatment, mood and quality of life.

The physiological effect of bowel cancer on nutrition is twofold. First, patients may have a reduced nutritional intake as a result of the obstructive nature of their disease. Surgery to relieve the obstruction is necessary in order for patients to tolerate enteral or oral nutrition. Second, malignant solid tumours can adversely affect metabolism, creating a syndrome called cancer cachexia, which is particularly common in advanced cancers. Unlike ordinary starvation where the body works to preserve its stores through reducing metabolic rate, a patient with cancer cachexia has an altered metabolism with increased turnover of protein, fatty acids and glycerol, and increased gluconeogenesis. This is thought to result from a systemic inflammatory response, with secretion of cytokines such as tumour necrosis factor α and interleukins 1 and 6, and changes in hormones with increased cortisol excretion and hyperinsulinaemia.

Cancer cachexia manifests as significant weight loss (10% or more of total body weight) particularly affecting lean body mass, anorexia and early satiety. The inflammatory response, changes in hormones and subsequent effect on metabolism make it difficult for patients to maintain or regain weight, even with nutritional support. There has been growing interest in trying to modify the inflammatory response through use of omega-3 (ω-3 or n-3) fatty acids (fish oils). Work to date has predominantly involved patients with pancreatic cancers and has shown that supplementing with n-3 fatty acids can positively affect weight, thereby improving quality of life (Davidson et al. 2004).

The treatment for bowel cancer can also adversely affect nutritional status. Surgery is the treatment of choice for colorectal cancer and nutritional status can affect outcome. Periods of being 'nil by mouth' or on limited oral fluids before and after surgery mean that suboptimal nutrition is received. Weight loss in surgical patients is associated with a higher incidence of both morbidity and mortality, and length of hospital admission is significantly shorter in well-nourished cancer patients (Bauer et al. 2002). Declining nutritional status is also often apparent in patients during radiotherapy treatment, and those with poor nutritional status tend to lose weight with each cycle of chemotherapy. It is therefore important to identify 'at-risk' colorectal cancer patients, ideally through routine screening for malnutrition, and initiate intervention using appropriate care pathways.

The effect of malnutrition on mood is well known, with declining nutritional status associated with increasing lethargy and low mood. Individual micronutrients have been linked with depression including B vitamins, thiamine and folate. Low selenium and zinc levels have also been associated with low mood. Iron deficiency anaemia is a common presenting symptom of colorectal cancer and associated with lethargy and poor concentration.

Nutritional management of the bowel cancer patient

Identifying malnutrition

Nutritional status can be identified in a variety of ways including weight history, body mass index (BMI), anthropometric measurements, nutrition risk index, subjective global assessment and nutrition screening tools using a combination of factors. Many nutritional screening tools have been developed but are often difficult to use and not always robustly tested. There has been a recent national initiative through the Malnutrition Advisory Group of the British Association of Parenteral and Enteral Nutrition (BAPEN) to develop a simple screening tool for malnutrition, which can be used across hospital and community settings (BAPEN 2004). The screening tool also provides basic care pathways, which can be adapted to suit individual environments and patient groups to ensure appropriate nutritional intervention is provided.

Even if a screening tool is not used, BAPEN recommends that, in addition to being weighed, all patients are asked the following questions in order to highlight any nutritional problems (Lennard-Jones et al. 1995):

- Have you unintentionally lost weight recently?
- Have you been eating less than normal?
- What is your normal weight?
- How tall are you?

Use of a nutritional screening tool is highly recommended for colorectal cancer patients in acute hospital and community settings. It is a simple way to ensure that nutritional status is monitored and appropriate nutritional intervention provided. Inclusion of a nutritional screening tool into integrated care pathways should be considered.

Nutritional support

Patients with a functioning gut who have or are at risk of poor nutrition should be given advice on adapting their normal diet to meet requirements (Barton et al. 2000). It is only if this is insufficient and treatment aims cannot be met through diet alone that prescribable supplements or enteral tube feeding should be considered. Unfortunately, inappropriate prescription of sip feeds is common, with lack of appropriate dietary advice being cited as the main reason (Gall et al. 2001). Providing dietary resources and training for doctors and nurses, particularly those in the community where access to a dietitian is often more limited, and establishing nutritional screening tools and care pathways may help to address this.

All patients who are prescribed sip feeds should have the aims of treatment clearly defined and receive regular monitoring, as compliance is often poor (Barton et al. 2000). Palatability of sip feeds is a common problem and is reported to be a cause of non-compliance. However, non-compliance may also be a reflection of reduced appetite rather than taste preference (McAlpine et al. 2003). When prescribed appropriately sip feeds can increase energy intake beyond that of normal food and promote weight gain with significant clinical benefits. This is particularly apparent in those with a BMI under 20 kg/m^2 (Stratton 2000). It is beneficial to use the skills of the dietitian to assess and advise patients on dietary manipulation and the use of prescribable supplements.

There is no evidence to support routine use of parenteral or enteral nutrition in well-nourished or mildly undernourished surgical patients, provided that significant oral nutrition is being consumed (Nitenberg and

Raynard 2000). If a protracted time without oral nutrition is anticipated, i.e. as a result of postoperative ileus, or a patient has significant weight loss or is underweight (BMI < 19 kg/m²), nutritional support should be considered. Decisions about artificial nutritional support should be multidisciplinary and include the dietitian. Many hospitals have a specialized nutrition support team (NST), made up of a dietitian, pharmacist, nutrition nurse specialist and clinician who advise on parenteral nutrition. Use of an NST has been shown to help rationalize use of parenteral nutrition, reduce infection risks and ensure that patients' nutritional requirements are safely met (Silk 1994).

Dietetic advice should be sought when considering enteral nutrition in malnourished patients with a functioning gut. Nasogastric tube feeding through a fine-bore feeding tube is the route of choice if short-term feeding is anticipated, i.e. < 4 weeks. If longer-term feeding is required, placement of a gastrostomy tube either endoscopically or under radiological guidance should be used. Patients can usually be discharged home on enteral nutrition with support from community nurses and dietitians.

Postoperative care

Many patients will be unable to meet their estimated nutritional requirements for some time postoperatively. Once patients can take free fluids they should be encouraged to include nourishing fluids. Many hospitals provide fortified soup, jelly and ice-cream, and some wards have instigated 'milkshake rounds' to help improve patients' nutritional intake. Both the dietitian and ward nurses have an important role in helping patients establish good oral nutrition. Nursing staff are on hand to encourage nourishing fluids and progression to diet, and can monitor nutritional status and intake. The dietitian can advise on specific dietary requirements, appropriate fluid and food, and use of any prescribable supplements. Once oral nutrition is established patients should be encouraged to eat as wide a variety of foods as can be tolerated, slowly increasing their intake of high-fibre foods.

Many patients are anxious about the reintroduction of diet after bowel surgery and have a limited understanding of digestion. Patients facing bowel surgery do not always have a good understanding of what part of the bowel is being removed, how this will impact on their digestive system and how faecal output will change. Without this knowledge explanation of any dietary changes and confidence in eating can be impaired. It is therefore important that those involved in treating and supporting the patient have a good understanding of the impact of surgery on nutrition and can confidently explain this in appropriate terms.

The basic role of the colon is to reabsorb water and sodium from the faecal fluid passing through the colonic lumen back into the blood-stream. Removal of the sigmoid or descending colon usually results in fairly solid, intermittent output, because much of the water has already been absorbed higher in the colon. Disease affecting the ascending or transverse colon often results in the need for a total colectomy and for-mation of an ileostomy, and the stool output is far more liquid and frequent. Although the bowel does adapt to some extent over time, this latter group of patients is at particular risk of electrolyte imbalance and dehydration.

Reduced absorption of nutrients is not normally a problem for patients undergoing colorectal surgery because both macro- and micronutrients are absorbed in the small intestine. Occasionally part of the terminal ileum may need to be removed and in patients who have no distal ileum vitamin B_{12} status should be monitored and supplemented appropriately.

Formation of a stoma can create dietary uncertainties, with patients often feeling that they need to follow a special diet. However, the general advice is for patients with stomas to resume a normal diet, including as wide a variety of foods as can be tolerated (Black 2000).

Formation of a colostomy preserves some colon, helping to ensure that water and sodium are adequately absorbed. Patients with a colostomy are encouraged to resume as near normal a diet as can be tolerated, but patients often modify their diet after surgery. A small study looked at dietary changes made by people with a colostomy 6 months after surgery. Few significant dietary changes were reported and changes that were made were primarily the result of improved appetite or avoiding unpleas-ant side effects. Most patients reported loose stools, but this was attributed to diet in only half of the patients (Bulman 2001).

Although the numbers were small, one can extrapolate that patients will often avoid a food only if the symptoms are unacceptable. If patients feel that a particular food causes a problem, encouragement should be given to retry it on a couple of occasions to establish that an individual food is the culprit. This helps to maintain as varied a diet as possible. Colostomy patients can also be prone to constipation so they should be encouraged to increase fibre intake slowly and take plenty of fluid. Eating regularly and including plenty of high-fibre foods can help faecal output become more formed and regulate bowel movements.

Formation of an ileostomy means that all fluid and sodium, alongside nutrients, need to be absorbed in the small intestine. The small intestine does adapt over time and absorption of water and sodium should improve. However, ileostomy patients should be advised to increase salt intake to replace gut losses and ensure adequate fluid to prevent dehy-dration. Often just adding salt at mealtimes, or including salty snacks such as crisps, yeast extract on bread or as a hot drink, is adequate (Black 2000). Patients should aim to take around 2 litres of fluid daily (around 8 cups of fluid) but this may need to be increased if the ileostomy output is high, the weather is very hot or the patient undertakes exercise. Sports drinks, diluted fruit juice or Coca-Cola (can be made flat if sugar is added, slowly!) might all be a useful way to replace fluid and electrolytes. If problems with electrolyte balance and dehydration persist, agents to slow down stoma output can be used, e.g. codeine, loperamide, and advice sought from the medical or nutrition team caring for the patient. Certain foods have been reported to increase diarrhoea in ileostomy patients including sorbitol, large amounts of fruit and vegetables, spicy food, fried food, chocolate and alcohol. Anecdotally, marshmallows, jelly, white rice, ripe bananas and stewed apple can help thicken stoma output.

Ileostomy patients should be reassured that stoma output colour and consistency will change depending on what is eaten and advised that food will often pass into the bag partially digested. The Ileostomy Association recommends that, after the initial postoperative phase, patients eat as wide a variety of foods as can be tolerated. Stoma obstruction can occur because the small bowel has a narrower lumen than the colon and ileostomy patients are often advised to avoid nuts, dried fruit, popcorn, mushrooms, sweetcorn, tough fruit and vegetable skins, and fibrous foods such as coconut or celery (Black 2000). Anecdotally, many ileostomy patients eat these foods without a problem and it would seem that chewing well, incorporating them as part of a meal and not taking large amounts of these foods help to improve tolerance. However, patients prone to obstruction or with a history of a small bowel stricture would be wise to take care with these foods and advice should be sought from the patient's stoma care nurse.

Ileostomy and colostomy patients both report problems with wind and odour. Suggestions for reducing wind production include avoiding brassica vegetables, beans and lentils, onions, spicy foods, fizzy drinks, lager or beer. Eating slowly and drinking peppermint tea may be helpful. Increased odour can sometimes be associated with eating fish, eggs or spicy foods. As before, patients should be encouraged to take a wide variety of foods and limit their diet only if the side effects are too difficult to cope with.

Although patients may require nutritional support and advice during hospital admission for surgery, many continue to struggle as outpatients. Indeed surgical patients have been reported to continue to lose weight up to 3 months postoperatively. It is therefore important to continue to monitor nutritional status and initiate appropriate intervention to support patients as in- and outpatients.

Nutrition and chemoradiation

Radiotherapy treatment in colorectal cancer is usually used only to treat rectal cancers. The side effects of treatment can include sickness, diarrhoea, increased tiredness, local skin reaction and sometimes inflammation of the bladder lining leading to cystitis. Chemotherapy can be used as adjunctive treatment to surgery or sometimes in palliation. Side effects are similar to radiotherapy including fatigue, diarrhoea, sickness, loss of appetite, taste changes and increased susceptibility to infections during the neutropenic phase of treatment. Patients who are malnourished before chemotherapy tend to lose weight with each cycle of chemotherapy. Response to chemotherapy treatment can be adversely affected by poor nutrition, with cachectic patients responding less well to chemotherapy treatment (Tisdale 1993).

Fatigue is often experienced by patients and can make buying and preparing food difficult. Practical support and ideas are needed. This can include buying ready-made meals or easy to prepare snacks, using friends and family to help, buying food on the internet or even considering temporary use of 'meals on wheels'.

Loss of appetite or early satiety is a common problem in patients undergoing treatment. Practical advice on adapting ordinary food to maximize nutrient density should be given, alongside the encouragement to eat frequent small meals or snacks, and take nourishing fluids if eating is difficult, e.g. milky drinks, homemade or commercially available milk shakes, smoothies or fortified soups. First-line dietary advice is often available from the local dietetic department or cancer unit, or from reputable sources such as CancerBACUP. Patients with significant weight loss or nutrition-related problems should be referred to a dietitian for further advice and possible introduction of appropriate prescribable supplements.

Nausea and vomiting can often be effectively controlled with medication and it is important to encourage patients to ask for medication to control these symptoms. High levels of serum calcium, altered liver function, constipation and bowel obstruction are all causes of nausea and vomiting in the colorectal cancer patient. It is important to remember that, in the context of cancer patients, there is no correlation between dietary calcium intake and serum calcium levels, so dietary restriction of calcium is of no benefit in patients with raised levels.

Some patients report increased sensitivity to smells or a persistent nausea that limits their ability to eat. Avoiding food smells by choosing cold rather than hot food and avoiding cooking or areas where food is being prepared is often helpful. Foods with a fresh taste or that have a dry texture are often better tolerated than high-fat, creamy or rich foods. Food or drink that contains ginger can also alleviate nausea. Eating little and often can be helpful and prevents becoming over-hungry, which can exacerbate nausea.

Taste changes can occur while having chemotherapy treatment with increased sensitivity to certain tastes, i.e. everything is very salty or sweet which can make it more difficult to find foods that are palatable. Some patients also report a complete lack of taste and consequently eating is not a pleasurable experience. Food aversions can also occur and have been reported in up to 56% of patients receiving chemotherapy (Mattes et al. 1992). Cancer patients commonly report avoidance of meat, coffee and chocolate, or instinctively avoiding foods that they ate before being sick. These patients should be reassured that taste changes and food aversions often occur, and support offered to find foods that they like, including advice on how to meet their nutritional requirements if intake is limited and encouragement to retry foods avoided at a later stage. Referring patients with significant problems to the dietitian, particularly one with specialist knowledge of cancer, can be helpful.

Mucositis can also occur after chemotherapy treatment. Good oral hygiene and adequate pain relief are important factors to consider. Helpful dietary hints include having soft foods with plenty of moisture, i.e. sauces, gravy, avoiding strongly flavoured or citrus-based foods, and avoiding foods at extreme temperatures, i.e. letting hot foods cool down and avoiding icy foods.

Patients undergoing chemotherapy will usually have periods of neutropenia, making them susceptible to infections, including food-borne ones. It is sensible to remind patients to use good food hygiene at home, and take care when eating out. High-risk foods such as raw eggs, unpasteurized dairy products or undercooked poultry should also be avoided during this period.

Diarrhoea and local skin reaction caused by radiotherapy can make it very painful to pass stools. Symptomatic advice is vital and modifying dietary intake may help. Patients are commonly advised to reduce fibre consumption if they have diarrhoea, the extent of which varies between radiotherapy units. It is important to emphasize that this is a short-term measure for symptomatic control and patients should be encouraged to reintroduce fibre slowly once the diarrhoea has stopped and they have recovered from treatment. To date there has been limited evidence to support the use of very-low-fat or lactose-free diets in patients undergoing pelvic radiotherapy. Dietetic supervision should be sought if these dietary restrictions are introduced, because it can be difficult to maintain adequate energy intake.

Cystitis can be a short-term problem for patients undergoing radio-therapy to their rectum. Encouraging patients to drink plenty of fluids is important and there is anecdotal evidence supporting the use of cranberry juice in patients with cystitis.

Prevention of recurrence of colorectal cancer

It is a logical deduction that diet could affect recurrence of colorectal can-cer. A large study (n = 1429) of individuals with previous colorectal adenoma investigated the impact of increased cereal fibre consumption on prevention of recurrent colorectal malignancy. Despite possible benefits of a high cereal fibre intake, modifying dietary fibre intake using wheat-bran fibre alone was not adequate to demonstrate a protective effect against recurrence of colorectal adenomas (Alberts et al. 2000). A further study (n = 2079) examined the impact of more complex dietary intervention on recurrence of colorectal adenomas. Unfortunately, the authors were unable to establish a positive association between following a low-fat, high-fibre diet high in fruit and vegetables and prevention of recurrence of colorectal adenocarcinoma. However, they could not conclude that a change in diet was of no benefit (Schatzkin et al. 2000).

Despite the lack of clinical trial evidence to date, it would seem pru-dent to advise patients who have fully recovered from treatment and have a good prognosis to follow current healthy eating advice, reducing total and saturated fat intake, increasing fibre, fruit and vegetable consumption to individual tolerance and encouragement to maintain a healthy weight (BMI between 19 and 25 kg/m^2).

Palliative care

Maximizing nutritional status is an important part of ensuring that patients have a good quality of life. However, it is important to set realis-tic expectations for patients and their carers about weight and nutritional intake. It is well recognized that carers and relatives are often far more concerned about weight loss and anorexia than patients at the end stages of their life, and nutritional treatment aims must be clear.

Eating and having a good appetite are an indication of health, and rel-atives can often feel that if they can get their loved one to eat or gain weight things would get better. The reality is that weight loss and poor appetite are usually part of the terminal phase of cancer and the appropriateness of aggressive nutritional intervention needs to be carefully discussed with the patient and the multidisciplinary team providing care. Enteral tube feeding in patients with functioning guts or parenteral nutrition in obstructed patients should be instigated only if ethical considerations have been discussed, and is clinically indicated, practically possible and most importantly what the patient wants.

Palliative chemotherapy in patients with locally advanced or metastatic colorectal cancer can be effective in reducing the rate of disease progression and prolonging survival. Cachectic patients respond less well to chemotherapy treatment, and some patients also have side effects from chemotherapy, which affect appetite, thus making nutritional support a necessary integral part of treatment (Tisdale 1993).

The emphasis of nutrition in palliative care has to be on maximizing nutritional status to help maintain a good quality of life. Monitoring of the patient's nutritional status needs to be undertaken with sensitivity, because it is not always appropriate to weigh patients if there is no intention to treat a deteriorating nutritional status. Symptom control is paramount if patients are to maximize their nutritional intake. Use of drugs to control symptoms of pain, nausea or altered bowel habits, coping strategies for fatigue, introduction of appetite stimulants such as megoestrol acetate, e.g. Megace, and steroids and treatment of depression can all help to improve nutritional intake (Wilcox et al. 1984, Karcic et al. 2002).

Specific dietary advice can also help with symptom control, e.g. increasing fibre and fluid intake for constipation, following a low-residue diet for diarrhoea or repeated bowel obstruction, having cold, plain food if nausea persists, or choosing foods that are moist or can be served with sauces if a dry mouth is a problem. Patients and relatives often find it helpful to have supportive, realistic advice to cope with symptoms of the disease and maximize nutritional intake. There may sometimes be a role for using prescribable sip feeds, but it is important to be clear about objectives for the use of these, taking into consideration patient preferences, compliance and quality of life.

It is also important to remember that eating is not just about maintaining nutritional status. Eating for enjoyment and social integration is vital for a good quality of life and should be remembered when providing nutritional advice and intervention.

Alternative diets

It is not uncommon for patients with cancer to want to try alternative or complementary diets in the hope of improving their chances of remission or cure. Increasing access to the internet has meant that patients are often overwhelmed with the nutritional advice available and are confused as to what they should do. Although many of these diets are supported by patient testimonials or anecdotal case studies, robust clinical evidence is usually lacking. Many dietary regimens require significant changes, which can sometimes be detrimental to nutritional status and often have financial implications.

Complementary and alternative diets usually share common themes, namely advising high fruit and vegetable consumption frequently raw or as juices, encouraging a high-fibre, low-fat intake, making them low in overall energy, restricting dairy products and encouraging vegetarian or vegan diets. Patients are often advised to buy organic produce and take megadoses of micronutrient supplements or other dietary products, but the clinical and financial benefits are often not convincingly proven. Alongside this the preparation for many of these diets is time-consuming and patients may feel guilty if they need to stop the diet for any reason.

In colorectal cancer patients these diets may be difficult to follow or inappropriate while recovering from surgery or undergoing chemotherapy or radiotherapy. Patients may not be able to regain or maintain weight if diets are low in fat, sugar and protein, whereas high fibre, fruit and vegetable consumption may increase diarrhoea or the risk of stoma obstruction.

Occasionally patients feel under pressure from relatives to follow alternative diets when in fact they would rather eat for enjoyment as well as health. In this group of patients a health-care professional can offer support in discussing diet with their relatives, allowing a patient's wishes to be recognized. However, it must also be remembered that patients often need to feel that they have some control and do something positive towards improving their health and 'fighting cancer'. Taking control of their diet and seeking out alternative or complementary regimens can provide some psychological benefit. The difficulty for health-care professionals involved in supporting cancer patients is being able to identify and understand which dietary practices are unsafe or put patients at nutritional risk, and to help them make informed choices about their nutritional intake. A dietitian, particularly one specializing in working with cancer patients, is well placed to advise, balancing the clinical safety of a diet and patient beliefs.

Summary of key points

- Certain dietary factors are implicated in the development of colorectal cancer or protection from the disease.
- Positive health promotion messages should encourage healthy lifestyle activities and the consumption of a diet low in fat and high in fibre, and acknowledge the 'five-a-day rule'.
- Malnutrition in cancer patients is multifactorial; however, the impact of nutritional status is far reaching, affecting morbidity and mortality.
- The use of a nutritional screening tool in hospital and community settings is highly recommended.
- Stoma formation can establish dietary uncertainties. Patients are encouraged to return to as near normal a diet as can be tolerated.
- The effects of chemoradiation are far reaching. Those patients with significant weight loss or other problems should be referred to a dietitian, preferably with specific expertise in this area.
- Some alternative and complementary dietary regimens require significant changes, can be detrimental to nutritional status and are expensive.

References

Alberts D, Martinez M, Roe D et al. (2000) Lack of effect of a high fibre cereal supplement on the recurrence of colorectal adenomas. New England Journal of Medicine 342: 16-62.

Barton A, Kay S, White G (2000) Managing people on sip feeds in the community. British Journal of Community Nursing 5: 541-2, 544, 546-7.

Bauer J, Capra S, Ferguson M (2002) Use of the scored Generated Subjective Global Assessment as a nutrition assessment tool in patients with cancer. European Journal of Clinical Nutrition 56: 779-85.

Black P (2000) Practical stoma care. Nursing Standard 14(41): 47-55.

British Association of Parenteral and Enteral Nutrition (BAPEN), Malnutrition Advisory Group (2004) The 'MUST' Report. Nutritional Screening of adults: a multidisciplinary responsibility. Executive Summary. Maidenhead: BAPEN.

Bulman J (2001) Changes in diet following the formation of a colostomy. British Journal of Nursing 10: 179-86.

Davidson W, Ash S, Capra S et al. (2004) The Cancer Cachexia Study Group. Clinical Nutrition 23: 239-47.

DeWys WD, Begg C, Lavin PT (1980) Prognostic effect of weight loss prior to chemotherapy in cancer patients. American Journal of Medicine 69: 491-7.

Doll R (1981) The causes of cancer: quantitative estimate of avoidance risks of cancer in the US today. Journal National Cancer Institute 66: 1191-308.

Gall MJ, Harner JE, Wanstall H (2001) Prescribing of oral nutritional supplements in Primary Care: can guidelines supported by education improve practice? Clinical Nutrition 20: 511-15.

Giovannucci E, Stampfer MJ, Colditz GA et al. (1993) Folate, methionine and alcohol intake and the risk of colorectal cancer. Journal of the National Cancer Institute 85: 875-83.

Karcic E, Philpot C, Morley JE (2002) Treating malnutrition with megestrol acetate: literature review and review of our experience. Journal Nutritional of Health Aging 6: 191-200.

Key T, Fraser G, Thorogood MV et al. (1999) Mortality of vegetarians and nonvegetarians: detailed findings from a collaborative analysis of 5 prospective studies. American Journal Clinical Nutrition 70(suppl 3): 516S-24S.

Lennard-Jones JE, Arrowsmith H, Davison C et al. (1995) Screening by nurses and junior doctors to detect malnutrition when patients are first assessed in hospital. Clinical Nutrition 14: 336-40.

McAlpine SJ, Harper J, McMurdo ME et al. (2003) Nutritional supplementation in older adults: pleasantness, preference and selection of sip feeds. British Journal of Health Psychology 8: 57-66.

Mattes DR, Curran WJ, Alavi J (1992) Clinical implications of learned food aversions in patients with cancer treated with chemotherapy or radiation treatment. Cancer 70: 192-200.

Nagengast FM, Grubben MJ, van Munster IP (1995) Role of bile acids in colorectal carcinogenesis. European Journal of Cancer 31A: 1067-70.

Nitenberg G, Raynard B (2000) Nutritional support of the cancer patient: issues and dilemmas. Critical Reviews in Oncology-Hematology 34: 37-68.

Schatzkin A, Lanza E, Corie D et al. (2000) Lack of effect of a low fat, high fibre diet on the recurrence of colorectal adenomas. New England Journal of Medicine 342: 1149-55.

Silk DBA (1994) Organisation of Nutritional Support in Hospitals. Maidenhead: BAPEN.

Stratton RJ (2000) Summary of a systematic review of oral nutritional supplement use in the community. Proceedings of the Nutrition Society 59: 469-76.

Tisdale MJ (1993) Cancer cachexia. Anticancer Drugs 4: 115-25.

Van Munster IP, Nagengast FM (1993) The role of carbohydrate fermentation in colon cancer prevention. Scandinavian Journal of Gastroenterology 200 (suppl): 80-6.

Wilcox JC, Corr J, Shaw J et al. (1984) Prednisolone as an appetite stimulant in patients with cancer. British Medical Journal 288: 27.

Will JC, Galuska DA, Vinicor F et al. (1998) Colorectal cancer: another complication of diabetes mellitus? American Journal Epidemiology 147: 816-25.

World Cancer Research Fund (1997) Food, Nutrition and the Prevention of Cancer: A global perspective. London: WCRF.

Further reading

Thomas B (ed.) (2001) Manual of Dietetic Practice, 3rd edn. London: Blackwell Science.

Useful website/contacts

www.bapen.org.uk

British Colostomy Association, 15 Station Road, Reading, Berks RG1 1LG. Tel: 0800 328 4257

CancerBACUP, 3 Bath Place, Rivington Street, London EC2A 3DR. Tel: 0909 8001234

Ileostomy and Internal Pouch Association, National Secretary, Peverill House, 1-5 Mill Road, Ballyclare, Co. Antrim, N. Ireland. Tel: 0800 0184724

Chapter 12

Professional issues

Ian Donaldson

In this chapter a number of challenges and responsibilities faced by health-care professionals are examined. The chapter starts with a consideration of professional accountability and ethical frameworks that can be applied to practice. Readers should note that legislation differs in each country and this chapter has been written from a perspective of English law. Three issues, each starting with a case study, are then examined. Each issue looks at legal, ethical and professional issues that the health-care professional needs to reflect upon. A consideration of both legal and ethical responsibilities is important because knowing what is the right thing to do requires drawing upon legal, ethical and professional perspectives.

Accountability

Accountability, or answerability, for one's professional practice is a key aspect of any professional's work. The ability to weigh up a situation and take the 'right' course of action based on professional judgement, experience and evidence base is the foundation for any professional's practice (the term 'right' has to be used with caution here and is not meant to imply a moral judgement, but that in the professional's clinical judgement that is the right action). We often consider being called to account in a negative way, in that something has gone wrong and individuals are called to account for their actions (such as the events surrounding the death of Wayne Jowatt at Queen's Medical Centre in 2001 – see Toft 2001). However, this really misses the point that, in a professional's daily work, he or she regularly has to make judgements and part of that process needs to be giving an explanation about why one course of action is preferred over another. Sometimes this debate is internal, because the individual considers his or her options, and at other times involves peers or the whole interprofessional team. Exercising one's accountability in most situations therefore does not occur in a vacuum and depends on a number of key factors. Although professional bodies such as the Nursing and Midwifery Council (NMC), the General Medical Council (GMC) and the Health Professions Council (HPC) would clearly argue that a registered professional is accountable for his or her actions, the context in which the individual works is important.

An essential but often overlooked precondition for accountability is that the individual not only has the ability to make a judgement but also has the necessary autonomy and authority to carry through any decision (Lee 1995). Dimond (2002) presents a simple but effective aide-mémoire for health-care professionals to remind them that they are accountable in four arenas: the public or state, the person, the employer and the professional body.

Accountability to the public

In this arena, accountability to current legislation is exercised. All professionals must be aware of their legal responsibilities and duties; ignorance of the law is no defence. Some legislation is relevant to any situation, e.g. the Health and Safety at Work Act and the Human Rights Act. Other legislation has specific links to health care such as the Access to Medical Records Act, the Coroner's Act and the Mental Health Act (soon to be revised). In this arena individuals are called to account in criminal courts for any breaches of legislation and are prosecuted by the Crown Prosecution Service (CPS). The balance of proof is that it is proven 'beyond reasonable doubt', and this standard is tested by an independent jury. Conviction may result in a fine and/or a custodial sentence.

Accountability to the person

In the UK certain laws are known as torts (Fletcher and Buka 1999). These are offences against the person and are seen in the realm of the civil courts. The term 'common law' or 'case law' is sometimes used because the laws are developed and refined through the courts. The current status of the law is recorded in cases. Particularly relevant examples are in consent law and clinical negligence (Montgomery 2003). A particular feature of English courts is a system of hierarchy where rulings made in a higher court are binding on lower courts. In complex and difficult cases the House of Lords and the Appeal Courts have the ultimate say in these matters when cases are heard. Key differences to criminal courts are that the balance of proof is 'on the balance of probabilities' and it is the individual him- or herself, the complainant, who brings the case to court through the legal representatives. If the courts find in favour of the complainant compensation is awarded. The level of compensation awarded depends on the level of damages and is further increased as a result of the rising legal costs in making claims. In 2001–2002 the NHS spent £446 million on clinical negligence, which includes defence costs and costs awarded to the claimants, prompting a review of the current situation in order to explore whether a new approach to managing such claims can be developed (Department of Health or DoH 2003a).

Accountability to the employer

All health professionals are contracted to work for their employer and as such are bound by the terms and conditions within their contract. A common clause is the need to maintain confidentiality and any breaches of contract may result in internal disciplinary action being taken, where the individual is required to give an account of his or her actions. A dilemma for some professionals here is where they feel their duties to the patient might be constrained by their duties to the employer. This demonstrates how even Dimond's simple model has to be interpreted because some situations cross-over and conflict with other arenas (Kohner 1996); some would say that this just reflects the complexity of professional life!

Accountability to the profession

All health-care professionals will be aware of their profession's code of conduct and, with the recent development of the Health Professions Council, most health-care professions are covered by a code of professional conduct. Each of the relevant councils can review any allegations of misconduct comparing the individual's actions against the set 'standards' in the code of conduct. It is a feature of a profession that self-regulation occurs, and, whereas in the other arenas it is a jury, the courts or a panel who assesses the situation, with professional accountability peers measure an individual's action. The professional bodies are then empowered with the right to remove a person from the register where cases of misconduct are proven.

The model for the arena of accountability represents the different places that are empowered to call the health professional to account. Clearly in some cases, such as Wayne Jowatt (Toft 2001), those individuals involved are called to account in all arenas.

The ethical framework described by Beauchamp and Childress (2001) is universally accepted and used within health care. The approach of principalism has its critics (Widdershoven 2002), and Beauchamp and Childress have attempted in the most recent edition of their book to reply to some of the criticisms by exploring in more detail the key virtues of professional practice. Central to their model are four principles of health care ethics:

- Respect for autonomy: the right of individuals to self-determination and therefore for health professionals to have a duty to empower and enable individuals to exercise their autonomy has a very strong emphasis in today's health-care world. There is a clear correlation between this principle and the laws of consent.

- Beneficence: actions should be aimed at bringing a benefit to the patient, sometimes known as 'best interests'; central to this is the individual's assessment of what lies in his or her best interests. Following the principle of beneficence without reference to the individual's perception lays the health professionals open to an accusation of paternalism.

- Non-maleficence: this principle reminds us that we should not inflict harm, but also that what is 'harm' requires a clear and detailed analysis in each context, e.g. harm caused by a course of chemotherapy may well be offset by the potential longer-term benefit of a cure.

- Justice: the fair allocation of resources, as opposed to retributive justice, is the final principle. Health-care professionals are in an ideal position to see the effect and may have to consider rationing and allocation of resources, and some high profile cases such as Child B (Montgomery 2003) have brought to the attention of both the public and the professions the need for clear and transparent criteria to be used when rationing decisions are made, and how the courts are being increasingly used to adjudicate in difficult decisions.

The second part of Beauchamp and Childress's (2001) ethical framework is the four ethical rules of confidentiality, privacy, veracity (to tell the truth) and fidelity. These rules are often enshrined within professional codes of conduct and are generally supported by appealing to the ethical principles and theories. However, as we see in the following sections that examine a number of clinical issues, sometimes it is not as clear as it would at first seem. Any moral deliberation requires not only the application of rules, principles and theories but also a clear understanding of the context of the situation (Randall and Downie 1996).

Confidentiality

Emily White is 73 years old. Her only family are a niece and a nephew who both live some distance away. Emily never married and has lived a very independent life, retiring from her work as an art historian for a national picture gallery 5 years ago when a sigmoid colectomy was performed after the discovery of a malignant tumour. She has been well until recent lower back and hip pain have brought her to her GP. A bone scan has revealed metastasis in the right hip and lumbar vertebrae. Her niece and nephew are very concerned and have been phoning the surgery wanting to know what is being done for Emily. However, Emily has specifically requested that neither be told the recent diagnosis.

In this case study the health-care professional's dilemma is whether to make a deliberate breach of confidentiality and if so on what grounds. This is quite distinct from an accidental breach where information is inadvertently released through, for example, an overheard conversation or records being left unattended, allowing someone who does not have any right access to the information. Accidental breaches should be prevented through systems being set up that protect information. The Data Protection Act of 1998 sets out eight principles, which should be applied to any information, whether electronic, or paper, to maintain privacy and confidentiality. The Human Rights Act 1998 further reinforces security of personal information as a right, where article 8 states the individual's right to 'respect of his private and family life, his home and his correspondence'. Alongside both these pieces of legislation are the Caldicott Guardians (DoH 2003b) whose role is to advise health professionals on confidentiality in NHS organizations. As well as confidentiality being an ethical rule, many argue that it is also justified by an appeal to the principle of respect for autonomy in that how we regard and manage information about people is a reflection of how we respect that person (Brown et al. 1997).

Most professional organizations make clear statements about practitioners' responsibilities towards protecting confidential information (the various professional groups' codes of conduct can be found on their respective websites – see Resources) and the importance of confidentiality is usually reiterated within the individual's contract of employment. Although legislation sets out rights and responsibilities, health-care professionals have to work in complex situations such as that described above. When reading about Emily many would already be considering what options might be possible and some would perhaps be asking more questions about the situation. What is the relationship between Emily and her relatives? How ill is she? Does she intend to tell her relatives herself? Essential to any approach to solving dilemmas such as these is that one takes a careful look at the situation before making any decision. Tschudin (1994) uses a simple model in which two questions are asked: 'What is happening?' and 'What is the fitting answer?' Logic says that the fitting answer cannot be found without first knowing what is happening. However, in many such scenarios what is the fitting answer is the first and only question asked and this can lead to the wrong course of action being taken.

The fact that patients can have control over information has to be accepted, but on what basis? Codes of conduct remind practitioners that they have a duty to preserve confidentiality and, under civil law, a patient could make a claim for damages where a health-care professional had breached confidentiality. Therefore, it is quite clear that breaches of confidentiality should be the exception rather than the rule. However, an unquestioning obedience to such a 'rule' would not always be in the best interests of those involved. Consider if Emily continued to deny any information to her family and how the situation could become very difficult to manage as her condition deteriorated. The use of professional judgement would need to come into play and, even within the legislation and codes of conducts already mentioned, a number of caveats can apply. Confidentiality can be breached when it is in the public interest. What constitutes the public interest can indeed be very difficult to define. Beauchamp and Childress (2001) present a useful model, which maps the probability of harm against the magnitude of harm. Cases where the magnitude of harm and probability of harm are high are situations that could be deemed to be in the public's interest. However, in Emily's case there is little likelihood of any public harm. What is less clear is how far a health professional can go in order to act in the patient's best interest. The principle of beneficence requires us to act in a way that is in the patient's best interest but has to be considered against what Emily thinks about the situation and balanced against the principle of non-maleficence.

It is at this point that we need to ask 'what is happening?' Without any consideration of this question, finding the fitting answer will be impossible. Emily may have requested that none of her family be told because she herself wanted to choose the right time and place. It might be that relationships in the family are strained and Emily does not want her family involved. Discussion between Emily and the team is therefore essential because what might transpire is a plan in which how information is to be shared is arranged. This of course is an ideal outcome, which respects

Emily's autonomy and would facilitate future working relationships, allow both Emily and her family to be effectively supported, and overcome a potentially very difficult situation to deal with.

What if this 'happy ending' cannot be achieved and Emily remains adamant that her family are not to be told? Working through this scenario, it is evident that Emily's request may place many of the team in a very difficult position and quite possibly would alienate the team from the family. Not an ideal situation when future care needs would need to be planned. Here the conflict between Emily's rights to control her own destiny and information about herself comes into conflict with the autonomy of individuals working within the team. It is recognized that a person cannot exercise his or her autonomy over another and in the case where a health professional could not maintain the standard of care to the patient he or she must be made aware of the tensions created. Mediation is a term that is frequently used but not often practised in situations such as Emily's, but it should be part of a health-care professional's repertoire to be able to negotiate the fitting answer with Emily.

Telling the truth

Case study

How much information should be given to a patient? Arthur has been admitted to a surgical ward with rectal bleeding. Before this episode of bleeding, which is his first, he had noticed a change in his bowel habits and some weight loss. Abdominal palpation reveals a mass in his left upper quadrant. The differential diagnosis includes a colonic tumour, which, with the history of altered bowel habit and weight loss, seems to be highly likely. Arthur has been very quiet after admission but following his family visiting he asks the staff 'what do you think is wrong with me?'. Initially the staff respond with 'we don't know and will have to wait for the tests', but he continues to ask every staff member with whom he comes into contact. Eventually some of the staff feel that he has to be told what the potential diagnosis might be; however, some disagree, saying that as we are not sure we should not worry him.

It is a common question that is asked: do patients have a right to know information about themselves? Tuckett (1999) suggests that there is some evidence that deception in health care is widespread. He clarifies this further by suggesting that in some cases practices range from telling semi-truths or avoiding telling (deception) to on occasions telling a deliberate lie. There are a number of potential arguments, which may be put forward to support not telling the truth. Each needs to be examined in order to explore whether they have any justification. It may be suggested that the patient does not want to know or as he or she has not requested any information, he or she is not interested. Clearly, in Arthur's case, this does not apply because he is asking questions. In some situations patients may state, in advance, that if there is any bad news they do not want to know. In these cases, which are extremely rare, great care is needed to ensure that the balance is kept between respecting an autonomous request and giving the patient information that they do need in order to understand and deal with what is happening to them. Beauchamp and Childress (2001) report on a number of studies that have been conducted showing that most individuals do want to know what is happening to them.

A second possible argument, which might be used in Arthur's and similar cases, is that one should pass on information to patients only when you are 'certain' of the facts. Whether one can ever know 'the whole truth' in some situations is questionable. However, the extreme opposite of this is to report to patients every suspicion, however tenuous and lacking in evidence. The dilemma for the health professional is to find a way between the two extremes of, on the one hand, not telling the patient anything, because one can never be certain of the truth, and, on the other, causing confusion and stress by informing the patient of every possibility, however unlikely.

The final possible argument to be used when justifying not telling the truth is benevolent deception. Proponents of this stance suggest that the harm (an appeal to the principle of non-maleficence) that could be caused when giving bad news or poor prognosis outweighs any obligation to tell the truth. The weakness of this argument is that it fails to ask what harm could be caused by leaving the patient in a state of not knowing. The impact on the therapeutic relationship, where those giving care are fully aware of the deception and seek to avoid situations where the patient could corner them, and the continued state of not knowing could in itself cause just as much harm. The other issue with this argument is that it is the basis on which patient confidentiality is frequently broken. How often do health professionals inform relatives of diagnosis and prognosis before the patient, on the grounds that they want to find out from the family how best to break the bad news? Arguably it is the patient who has the right to this information and the right to request that it is kept in confidence, but the outcome of this well-meaning 'fact finding' is often to create the final argument for not telling the truth. So often, conflict occurs when the family request that the information be withheld on the basis of the distress it would cause to the patient. Such conflicts are best avoided because they can affect working relationships with the family who feel that the health-care team have ignored their wishes when it is decided to tell the patient the truth.

Ethically the practice of avoiding telling the patient the truth has to be questioned on three counts. It undermines patient autonomy, because without the information the patient is unable to make any decisions about treatment and care. This has profound implications for consent, because without the information the patient cannot give informed consent and in some cases may argue that any consent gained was invalid; some would argue that this treats the patient as a means to someone else's ends. The second argument is that there is an implicit promise between the patient and health-care professionals to tell the truth. When communicating with others in helping relationships it is usually expected that the exchange will be truthful; for it to be otherwise calls into question the motives of the individual. Furthermore in Arthur's case he has submitted himself for investigations with, one would expect, the understanding that the test results will be shared with him. The third argument revolves around trust, an important foundation of any relationship, let alone a professional relationship. Rogers (2002) points out that doctors and other health-care professionals have to trust patients to give accurate information in order to make a diagnosis and evaluate the effectiveness of treatments. Therefore the question that has to be asked is whether trust can be one-sided and whether the patients themselves are not expecting health-care professionals to be open and honest with them.

If despite direct questioning Arthur does not get any truthful answers to his questions, his trust in the health team will deteriorate and he will be disempowered. The therapeutic relationship will be difficult to maintain at any level and with any professional because Arthur's 'experience' will be that you cannot trust anyone. Perhaps the other aspect of this scenario, which also requires consideration, is how the team works. This type of scenario can often bring team members into conflict when opposing or different courses of action are preferred. Randall and Downie (1996) point out that often the consensus model is not an effective one to follow because it tends to bring those with opposing values into conflict and then sight of the patient's needs is lost. Some may argue that this is what has happened with Arthur and that, when asking the reflexive question 'what is happening?', they recognize that Arthur's needs are being submerged by others. It might be the family or a member of the team who has requested that he is not told or it might be some unwritten 'protocol' that releasing this information is done by one individual or group. These aspects can and should be examined before such a situation as Arthur is in occurs. Questions such as when to tell, what to tell, how to tell and who should tell the truth are the ones that need to be addressed.

Consent and treatment decisions

Case study

Martin has just had a left hemicolectomy for a tumour. He is a self-employed financial adviser. After the surgery and the pathologist's report, he is advised to undergo a course of chemotherapy. Martin is very unsure about what to do and requests time and further information to make his decision. He has stated to a number of the team that he has had enough and does not want to be 'messed around' anymore.

In Martin's case respect for autonomy and the law of consent and refusal take centre stage. Respect for autonomy plays a very important part in health-care ethics. Although Beauchamp and Childress (2001) do not suggest that it is the most important principle in current society, great value is placed on the rights of the individual and one of the rights, to make decisions about oneself, is very highly valued. Gillon (1986, p. 60) defines autonomy as:

> The capacity to think, decide, and act on the basis of such thought and decision freely and independently and without let or hindrance.

The law is clear about an individual's rights to give and refuse consent (Montgomery 2003), providing he or she is an adult and mentally competent. The Family Law Reform Act 1969 permits 16-year-olds to give consent and the Gillick case (Montgomery 2003) permits children to give consent, providing the child has sufficient understanding. In Martin's case, consent will need to be obtained for any further treatment such as chemotherapy; he is an adult and under UK law all adults are presumed competent unless proven otherwise.

An essential prerequisite for an autonomous choice to be made is that certain preconditions are met. These are being able to understand the circumstances, able to make rational choices and finally able to act on such choices without any coercion. Without access to and the ability to understand information that pertains to the circumstances, an autonomous decision cannot be made. The importance of having this information further strengthens the argument for telling the truth and also reminds health professionals that it is not enough to give the information but to give it in a way that is understandable. The link here is to the ethical ideal of informed consent. Some refer to it as an ideal, because it is not always achieved, although the NMC and GMC strongly support the notion of consent being fully informed. To understand the information alone is not, however, sufficient.

Two other pre-conditions need to be met so that the individual has the mental capacity to weigh up this information, i.e. to make a rational choice. We must be clear that the term 'rational' means that the individual is able to consider the information and reach a reasoned decision, rather than reach the same decision as that 'preferred' by the team, e.g. Martin may have been informed that his cancer had spread to both his liver and his spine and that any chemotherapy would only delay rather than halt the progression of his disease. Coupled with a fear of needles one can see how a rational decision could be to refuse any further treatment. However, if the prognosis is significantly different, it would be relevant to check on Martin's understanding of the context of the situation, because to refuse a treatment that had a high degree of success could be construed as irrational. Once again we see how important it is to understand what is happening, but similarly health professionals have to be careful that they do not abandon their patients to some misguided sense of autonomy; just because the patient says that he or she does not want something does not mean that staff should immediately follow without first being certain that the decision is autonomous.

We can link this discussion to the legal position and case law surrounding consent and refusal. Two key cases are cited in such situations: *Re C (Adult)* and *Re B* (Commentary 2002, Montgomery 2003). In both cases questions were raised as to whether the patient was competent and able to refuse treatment (in *Re C*'s case it was a below-knee amputation and in *Re B* it was a refusal to continue with ventilation after paralysis from the neck down). In both cases refusal was seen as placing the individual's life in jeopardy and questions were asked as to whether the individual understood the gravity of the situation and also whether the individual had the necessary mental capacity to weigh up the information and arrive at a rational decision. The case law is now established that refusal is the right of any mentally competent adult and that mental capacity is established by considering two aspects:

1. Is the patient able to comprehend and retain information, especially the likely consequences of any action?
2. Is the patient able to use this information and to weigh it up as part of the process of arriving at a decision?

An answer in the affirmative to both questions confirms that the patient has the necessary capacity to make a decision and any refusal should be recognized.

In returning to our case, the question has to be 'is Martin mentally competent?' Although English law is clear that the presumption should be that he is mentally competent, it is useful for those caring for him to understand how mental capacity would be tested in an English court. There is, however, one further question that has both a legal and an ethical aspect and is a precondition for autonomy. Is the individual free from controlling influences? Making decisions such as that faced by Martin can place great strains on the individual and there is potential for others, both family and health professionals, to overly influence his decision. The courts recognize that decisions made under undue influence (*Re T*) can be overridden by the team acting on the basis of what is in the individual's best interests.

In returning to Martin's case, once again it is clear that the most appropriate response is to ensure that he has the necessary information and space in order to reach his own decision. Those giving the information do have to tread the fine line between ensuring that he has all the information, the risks, benefits and alternatives; it has to be done in a way that does not place any pressure or be overly directive. Exploring with him his concerns and dealing with those issues are also a key role of the caring health professional who is working towards promoting Martin's autonomy.

Conclusion

In looking at these three cases we can see that you cannot ignore the ethical, legal and professional domains. In many cases the law supports what is seen as the ethically right decision, but equally there are many instances where there is less certainty. This, some would argue, is the 'swampy lowlands' of practice which need to be worked through and without doubt one must accept that, in each of the cases reviewed, a different outcome may be argued were the situations or contexts to change. This reminds us that much of our professional decision-making, although underpinned by law, ethics and codes of conduct, is heavily influenced by the context of the situation. It is also a reminder to all practitioners that a failure to ask what is happening will not lead them to the fitting answer.

Summary of key points

- Personal accountability is a key aspect of all health professionals' work.
- Professional decision-making is underpinned by knowledge of the law, ethics and codes of conduct.
- The law is in a state of constant change and a health professional is required to be aware of the current legislation that is relevant to his or her country.
- What is legally right may not always be the ethically right thing to do and vice versa.
- An understanding of ethical principles and the facts of any situation are vital to ensure that any action taken is based on a sound examination of all the relevant issues.

References

Beauchamp T, Childress J (2001) Principles of Biomedical Ethics, 5th edn. Oxford: Oxford University Press.
Brown J, Kitson A, McKnight T (1997) Challenges in Caring: Explorations in nursing and ethics. Cheltenham: Stanley Thorne.
Commentary (2002) Competent adult patient: the right to refuse life sustaining treatment. Medical Law Review 10: 210-26.
Department of Health (2000) An Organisation with a Memory: Report of an expert group on learning from adverse events in the NHS. London: The Stationery Office.
Department of Health (2003a) Making Amends - Clinical negligence reform. London: Department of Health.
Department of Health (2003b) Confidentiality: NHS Code of Practice. London: Department of Health.
Dimond B (2002) Legal Aspects of Nursing, 3rd edn. Harlow: Longman.
Fletcher L, Buka P (1999) A Legal Framework for Caring. Basingstoke: Macmillan.
Gillon R (1986) Philosophical Medical Ethics. Chichester: John Wiley & Sons.
Kohner N (1996) The Moral Maze of Practice: A stimulus for reflection and discussion. London: King's Fund.
Lee R (1995) Resources and professional accountability In: Tingle J, Cribb A (eds), Nursing Law and Ethics. Oxford: Blackwell.
Montgomery J (2003) Health Care Law, 2nd edn. Oxford: Oxford University Press.
Randall F, Downie R (1996) Palliative Care Ethics: A good companion. Oxford: Oxford University Press.
Rogers W (2002) Is there a moral duty for doctors to trust patients? Journal of Medical Ethics 28(2): 77-80.
Toft B (2001) External inquiry into the adverse incident that occurred at Queen's Medical Centre Nottingham 4 January 2001. London: Department of Health; available at: www.publications.doh.gov.uk/qmcinquiry/index.htm.
Tschudin V (1994) Deciding Ethically. London: Baillière Tindall.
Tuckett A (1999) Nursing practice: compassionate deception and the good Samaritan. Nursing Ethics 6: 383-9.
Widdershoven G (2002) Alternatives to principalism: phenomenology, deconstruction and hermeneutics. In: Fulford K, Dickenson D, Murry T (eds), Healthcare Ethics and Human Values. Oxford: Blackwell.

Table of cases

Re B (Adult: Refusal of Medical Treatment) [2002] 2 All ER 449
Re C (Adult) (Refusal of Treatment) [1999] 1 WLR 290
Re T (Adult: Refusal of Treatment) [1992] 4 All ER 649

Resources: websites related to professional regulation

General Medical Council: www.gmc-uk.org/index.htm
General Social Care Council: www.gscc.org.uk/index.asp
Health Professions Council: www.hpc-uk.org/index.html
Nursing and Midwifery Council: www.nmc-uk.org/nmc/main/home.html

Chapter 13

Complementary therapies and cancer

Helen Gandhi

Cancer is one of the most prevalent diseases in modern society with one in three people in the UK being diagnosed with cancer in their lifetime; of those one in four people will die from the disease. Some cancers are more easily treated than others.

The main orthodox cancer treatments are surgery, radiotherapy, chemotherapy and combination therapy. At times these can appear to be invasive, painful and dehumanizing for patients (De Valois 2003).

It is reported that cancer patients frequently turn towards complementary therapies, their perception being that these have the non-toxic effect, the 'feel good factor' (Wilkinson 2002). Patients are not necessarily in search of a 'cure', but seeking wholeness and healing (Wright 2004). Studies conducted by Weil and Rees (2001) and Lewith (2002) identified that over 30% of people with cancer used complementary therapies. Indeed, the Bristol Cancer Help Centre UK pioneered the holistic approach to cancer care, and successful integration of complementary therapies, in the early 1980s. Initially surrounded by scepticism, this approach is now increasingly incorporated into mainstream health care (Wright 2004). Professor Richards' preface in the *National Guidelines for the Use of Complementary Therapies in Supportive and Palliative Care* acknowledged that there is a substantial number of patients who receive complementary therapies alongside mainstream treatment (Tavares 2003).

A recent report from the House of Lords' Select Committee on Science and Technology (Ernst 1999) recognized that complementary therapy is widely used and its popularity continues to rise. In spite of the limited data available, it has also highlighted the failure of surveys to consider the increased use of self-medication by the general public of over-the-counter remedies such as analgesics, cough medicines, antacids and vitamins.

Why people turn to complementary therapies is not fully understood, although many opinions and theories are proposed (Furnham 1996). Regardless of the lack of documentary evidence, Brewer (1989) believes the achievement of a complementary approach to be tangible and direct.

Several factors have been highlighted for the growing interest in complementary and alternative (CAM) therapies among health consumers. Based on available literature Stone (1999, pp. 46–50) suggests the following reasons:

- Fear of professionals
- Disaffection/mistrust of conventional medical practitioners
- Disillusionment with orthodox medicines that never fulfil their promise
- Being treated with respect and as an educated consumer
- Perception of competence and satisfaction with practitioners
- Experimentation, openness to experience and shopping for health
- Patients'/consumers' rights' movements
- Change in zeitgeist (ideas and spirit of time: the ideas prevalent in a period and place, particularly as expressed in literature, philosophy and religion).

Within the National Health Service (NHS) in the UK, almost all cancer centres, hospices and units offer some form of complementary therapy with palliative care being at the forefront of incorporating complementary therapies into orthodox care (Gray 2000). Hospice and palliative care centres were among the first health-care establishments in Britain to welcome aromatherapy as a possible mode of relief to their patients (Price and Price 1995). Palliative/supportive care and complementary therapy are two movements that have grown in parallel and are now recognized as an important part of good practice in the management of cancer care (Cawthorn and Carter 2000). The report of the Expert Advisory Group on Cancer (1995) (*The Calman–Hine Report*) recognized complementary therapies as an essential component of best practice in cancer care, alongside areas such as effective communication, information giving and psychosocial support.

Within the UK the most popular therapies include aromatherapy, reflexology, relaxation, massage and meditation (Macmillan Cancer Relief 2002).

Definition

Based on the complex nature and dissimilarity between alternative and complementary therapies, an appropriate definition is difficult to provide. Generally, the term 'complementary therapies' infers those treatments that may be used simultaneously and in combination with orthodox medical treatment (Beech 2001). Complementary medicine is described by the World Health Organization (WHO) as those types of medicine usually placed beyond the official health sector (WHO 1986). Trevelyan and Booth (1994) argue that this definition can jeopardize well-established therapies because it includes those thought to be more suspect and supports the significance of West's (1994) categorization of therapies. Therapies in this instance are divided into different types, namely those based on a degree of skill, professionalism and training, in comparison with do-it-yourself and self-care techniques. More recently Professor Ernst prepared, for the House of Lords, the following definition (Ernst 1999, p. 3):

> Complementary medicine is diagnosis, treatment and/or prevention which complements mainstream medicine by contributing to a common whole, by satisfying a demand not met by orthodoxy or by diversifying the conceptual frameworks of medicine.

Historical background

Many of the therapies currently seen as complementary or alternative were in the past considered to be traditional before the development of modern medicine (Stevenson 1997). Greek and Roman physicians viewed massage as the principal way of healing suffering and pain relief. In the fifth century BC, Hippocrates, the father of medicine, attempted to stem the spread of the plague in Athens with aromatic fumigation of the streets (Arcier 1990).

Essences were used in the eighteenth century to control the spread of disease. A familiar preparation was the 'four thieves' vinegar, which consisted of absinthe, rosemary, lavender, sage, mint, cinnamon, nutmeg, garlic and camphor macerated in vinegar. This remedy was applied all over the body to fight against infection (Arcier 1990).

Homoeopathy's history can also be traced back to Hippocrates who first developed the idea that an agent that can cause a disease might also be used to treat it (Trevelyan and Booth 1994).

The origins of reflexology date back to early Egyptian times, evidenced by inscriptions found in a physician's tomb (Byers 1983).

Nursing and complementary therapy

Since the 1980s there has been an increasing integration of complementary therapies into mainstream services (Mantle 1997), with a growing number of health professionals incorporating complementary therapies into their practice. The exact numbers are unknown because few data are available (Beech 2001). The tactile therapies, such as aromatherapy, reflexology and massage, are the kinds primarily used by professionals (Rankin-Box 1997). The reasons for this combination of therapies within nursing are complex. Trevelyan and Booth (1994) suggest this may be the result of changes in nurse education and the reduction in time spent on 'hands-on' care. It could also be argued that nurses are drawn towards CAM because this offers a holistic approach to patient care, supporting autonomous practice with an increasing scope for expansion and integration into patient care. Additional benefits include independence, decision-making and taking action.

Combining complementary therapies with practice raises a number of issues and concerns, with implications for the individual professional (see Chapter 12). Each has a duty of care to promote safety and efficacy towards their patients, the responsibility resting entirely with the practitioner, who should ensure that he or she has the evidence to support the safety or otherwise of the specific therapy. As a result of a lack of research some therapies have unproven effectiveness (Tavares 2003).

McVey (2000) highlights the nurses' ethical and professional responsibility to the patient, who is protected by the United Kingdom Central Council (UKCC; now the Nursing and Midwifery Council or NMC). It is the nurses' responsibility to ensure that introduction of any CAM is done so with full cooperation from the line manager and trust/institution protocols, ensuring that guidelines with a robust audit system are in place. Unless specifically negotiated, it is unlikely that CAM is encompassed within the contractual agreement of employment, leaving the health professional in a vulnerable position (Stone 1999). Another major concern relates to training and patient protection. Is the practitioner who is using complementary therapies competent to do so? There are many courses available in complementary therapy, with varying training standards depending on the particular therapy (Stevenson 1997). The professional who considers integrating complementary medicine needs to maintain the standards upheld by his or her professional body, e.g. the NMC. As with conventional medicine, complementary medicine is safe only if practised by suitably qualified, competent practitioners, and it can be harmful in unskilled hands. Attendance at a 1- or 2-day course on CAM does not qualify a health professional to administer therapies.

Guidelines for the use of complementary therapies are mentioned in the UKCC's document, *On Standards for the Administration of Medicines*, and state that the use of complementary therapies should be 'based on sound principles, available knowledge and skill' (UKCC 1992b) (see Chapter 12 for further details on professional issues).

Patient expectations should not be raised about disease cures and patients should be made aware that the aims of therapies are to offer additional support, enhance the quality of life and provide symptomatic relief. 'Patients should be encouraged to accept all appropriate forms of treatment, including conventional treatments' (Stevenson 1996, cited in Gray 2000, p. 79).

Professionals are also advised to check that their public liability indemnity insurance includes the appropriate practised therapy (see Chapter 12). Organizations such as the Royal College of Nursing (RCN) can supply a list of the therapies covered.

McVey (2000) noted that national guidelines for determining the practice of complementary therapies were insignificant. This situation has now changed since the 2003 publication of *National Guidelines for the Use of Complementary Therapies in Supportive and Palliative Care* by the Prince of Wales Foundation for Integrated Health. The foundation was established at the personal initiative and involvement of His Royal Highness the Prince of Wales. The aim of the foundation in terms of research into complementary medicine is the development of health-care institutions and professionals in order to achieve the Prince of Wales's vision of integrated health care in the twenty-first century (Anon 2002, p. 54).

Six keys principles underpin this work (Prince of Wales Foundation for Integrated Health 2003):

1. Promotion of a holistic and integrated approach to health care
2. Emphasis on the key importance of individuals taking more responsibility for their own health care
3. Acknowledgement of the intrinsic healing capacity of every person and awareness that different approaches and interventions may need to be employed together to restore health and well-being
4. Establishment of an evidence base for integrated health care
5. Acceptance that every person should have access to the treatment approach of his or her choice
6. Acceptance that the public has a right to expect health-care services to be provided by appropriately educated, safe, competent and regulated practitioners.

Complementary therapies

Unlike conventional medicine and its disease-oriented approach, complementary medicine focuses on health and healing. Patients are viewed as 'whole beings' with minds and spirits; therapies aspire to enhance or stimulate the body's self-healing capacities (Fulder 1988). The phrase 'complementary therapies' encompasses the more familiar such as acupuncture to the obscure.

Nine therapies that are widely used in palliative and supportive care were reviewed for their perceived beneficial effects. Those now recognized are listed in the *National Guidelines for the Use of Complementary Therapies in Supportive and Palliative Care* (Tavares 2003). Guidance is also given on the precautions and contraindications when used in this context.

Therapies reviewed

- Touch therapies: massage, aromatherapy and reflexology.
- Healing and energy therapies: reiki, spiritual healing and therapeutic touch
- A third group consisting of: hypnosis and hypnotherapy, acupuncture and homoeopathy.

Aromatherapy and therapeutic massage

Aromatherapy is one of the most widely used therapies in palliative support and a report from the House of Lords (Ernst 1999) into complementary health practices acknowledged the value of aromatherapy in palliative care.

Aromatherapy is defined as: 'the use of essential oils to promote health and vitality of the body, mind and spirit by inhalations, baths, compresses, topical application and massage' (Price 1985, p. 213).

Essential oils are a plant's 'life force' and are secreted from the cells, ducts and glands of the plant, collected by a variety of methods such as distillation. Essential oil is present in every part of the plant, including the roots, barks and leaves (Price 1987).

The most popular use of aromatherapy is through massage; the use of oils is said to enhance the effects of massage therapy (Wilkinson 2002). These oils can also be used in vaporizers, baths creams and lotions.

Massage

Massage may be defined as any systematic form of touch, which has been found to give comfort or promote good health (Maxwell-Hudson 1990). This is a generic term used for a variety of techniques, which involve touching, pressing, kneading and manipulation of the body's soft tissues for therapeutic purposes (Calvert 2003, Jackson 2003). Massage is the basis of many therapies such as acupuncture, aromatherapy and reflexology (Trevelyan and Booth 1994). Touch is one of the first human senses to develop and the most highly used. It is a basic behavioural need and its importance for both mental and physical health has been widely researched (Montague 1986). Providing our need for touch is satisfied we grow healthily, but, should this be inhibited, normal development may be impaired. Massage is a sharing of touch, placing hands on the body, head or feet (Lidell et al. 1990).

Therapeutic massage with or without aromatherapy oils has both a physical and a psychological effect, relieving stress, anxiety and tension, while promoting a sense of well-being.

The use of massage in cancer is often questioned, assumptions being made that this technique can disseminate disease to other parts of the body. Scientific evidence to prove or disprove these queries is lacking (Kassab and Stevenson 1996). This opinion is supported by McNamara (1997) who, after carrying out a study from the Wandsworth Cancer Centre, concluded that there is also 'nothing to show that it does not'. Gentle massage, according to Tissarand and Balacs (1995), is probably no more dangerous in cancer sufferers than gentle exercise, walking or taking a bath.

The aromatherapist needs to be aware of the benefits as well as the contraindications and precautions when using massage with patients undergoing cancer treatments.

History taking is an essential part of a patient's treatment. Massage therapists, aromatherapists and reflexologists are trained to assess and screen patients, taking into consideration other factors such as medication, nutrition and lifestyle. Normally an hour of a patient's time is required to undertake an assessment.

The benefits of aromatherapy and therapeutic massage are many, both physical and psychological; however, assessment of any physical benefits is easier to establish than that for psychological ones. Massage improves the circulation of blood and lymph and can slow down the pulse rate, and claims that blood pressure can be reduced have been reported (Price and Price 1995).

The psychological benefits, although difficult to evaluate, suggest that they play a part in the holistic healing effect by:

> Relaxing an apprehensive mind, uplifting depression and despair, relieving panic or anger and importantly giving a person the feeling that someone cares enough to spend time . . .

> Price and Price (1995, p. 94)

Contraindications and precautions

- Do not massage over a cancer site, avoiding any direct pressure on the area of the cancer.
- Dilution of the oil is important. Patients undergoing chemotherapy may be sensitive to smells. Dilution should be to 0.5% (Price and Price 1995).
- Do not massage over a surgical wound, and avoid stoma sites, cannulae and fracture sites.
- Avoid a limb or foot with suspected or diagnosis of deep vein thrombosis.
- Do not massage if the patient has an infection or temperature (adhere to policies and guidelines for infection control).
- Do not massage patients with a low platelet count; a low count causes a patient to bruise more easily.
- Gentle massage can be administered to those areas of the body not affected by cancer, such as the hands, face or feet as these are non-invasive procedures that can be tailored to suit patient tolerance.
- Therapists based in the hospital setting should ideally practise in a separate room and not in the ward area. Note that special consideration must be given to the use of vaporizers, especially when used in an area where some patients may have respiratory conditions or are sensitive to smells. The dilution of the oils can be further reduced in situations where there is a tendency for smell sensitivity. Record keeping of any given treatment should be in accordance with local policy.
- Radiotherapy considerations include awareness of possible side effects, such as fatigue, soreness of skin and digestive disturbance. Entry and exit sites should be avoided during and 3-6 weeks after treatment (Tavares 2003).
- Medical permission may be required in some instances.
- Signed patient consent must be obtained before commencing treatment.

This list was adapted from the *National Guidelines for the Use of Complementary Therapies in Supportive and Palliative Care* (Tavares 2003).

Reflexology or zone therapy

The history of reflexology dates back thousands of years. Information acquired from ancient texts, illustrations and artefacts validates that reflexology was practised by Egyptian, Chinese, Japanese, Indian and Russian communities (Norman and Cowan 1988).

Reflexology is a method used for activating the body's own powers of healing (Norman and Cowan 1988) and is defined by Byers (1983) as a science that deals with the principle of energy zones in the feet and hands which correspond to all the glands, organs and parts of the body. This technique is a unique means of using the thumb and fingers on specific reflex areas (Byers 1983, p. 11):

1. To relieve stress and tension
2. To improve blood supply and promote the unblocking of nerve impulses
3. To help nature achieve homoeostasis.

A reflexologist should never diagnose or treat a specific condition; the potential effects of treatment are to alleviate physical and emotional symptoms (Lynn 1996).

Reiki

Dr Mikao Usui rediscovered this ancient method of healing in Japan in the 1800s. The goal of reiki (pronounced ray-key and from the Japanese word meaning universal energy) is to restore balance in mind, body and spirit to improve well-being, working to redress any imbalance within these areas (Tavares 2003).

Treatment usually involves the therapist placing his or her hands in 12 different positions: four on the head, four on the front of the body and four on all major organs and glands. By treating the whole body, reiki aims to heal the reason for the disease and imbalance, including the symptoms.

Spiritual healing

Spiritual healing (often referred to as healing) is a process that promotes better health by channelling the healing energies of the healer to the patient (National Federation of Spiritual Healers 1998). Healing often assists the speed and extent of recovery from serious illness, major surgery or the effect of treatments such as chemotherapy and radiation therapy. It complements conventional medicine (National Federation of Spiritual Healers 2003). There is little evidence to support spiritual healing; however, this method remains popular in supportive and palliative care (Macmillan Cancer Relief 2002).

Acupuncture or 'needle piercing'

Very fine needles are inserted into the skin to stimulate specific points called acu-points. It has traditionally been taught as a preventive form of health care, but when used in the treatment of a variety of acute and chronic conditions benefits have been noted. In 1980 the WHO issued a list of diseases where acupuncture is known to be effective (Tue 1999, p. 203).

Acupuncture has been used for over 3000 years in China as a major part of their primary health-care system. In modern times, it is used for the prevention and treatment of disease; to strengthen the immune system, particularly at seasonal changes when colds and influenza are more prevalent; to relieve pain; and also in surgery as an anaesthetic. Acupuncture as an adjunct to conventional medicine is considered an appropriate management option in palliative care; evidence to support its use as a curative treatment for cancer has not yet been validated (British Medical Acupuncture Society 2003). Techniques in which any substance is injected through a hollow needle into the skin are not considered to be acupuncture; equally treatments that do not include piercing the skin are not a recognized procedure.

Acupressure

Based on the principles of acupuncture, this ancient Chinese technique involves the use of finger pressure (rather than needles) at specific points along the body. It is used to treat common ailments such as arthritis, tension and stress, aches and pains, and menstrual cramps. This technique can be applied in general preventive health care, e.g. Acubands applied to pressure points on the wrist for the prevention of nausea associated with motion sickness or chemotherapy.

Therapeutic touch

Developed in the 1970s by Dolores Krieger, a Professor of Nursing at New York University, therapeutic touch (TT) is a process by which energy is transmitted from one person to another for the purpose of stimulating the healing process of one who is ill or injured (Egan 1992). Despite its name, TT rarely involves physical contact between practitioner and patient. It involves simply placing or laying on of hands on to or in close proximity to the person to be healed. The intention of the practitioner carrying out this process is to assist with healing of the person involved. Usually the procedure takes between 10 and 15 minutes (Krieger 1975, p. 21).

The procedure consists of the practitioner moving hands in a rhythmic, downward movement, maintaining a short distance from the body of the client, working downwards from the head towards the feet. While carrying out the procedure the patient is continuously assessed for any imbalances in the energy field. When a 'blocked' area is discovered, the practitioner will focus on this area. A flowing movement is used, starting at the top of the site located and downwards away from the body. This procedure is repeated until the practitioner is satisfied that the blockage has been cleared. After treatment patients can experience a feeling of deep relaxation (Tavares 2003).

Hypnosis and hypnotherapy

Clinical hypnotherapy means applying hypnosis to treat a variety of medical and psychological problems. Hypnosis has been described as a psychological state in which certain human capacities are heightened whereas others fade into the background. (Tavares 2003). Usually people receiving therapy experience a sense of deep relaxation, their attention being narrowed down, and focused on appropriate suggestions made by the therapist (Douglas 2003).

Homoeopathy

The word homoeopathy is derived from the Greek word 'homoeos' meaning like or similar and 'pathos' meaning suffering. Samuel Hahnemann, a German doctor in the eighteenth century, established homoeopathy based on the principle that 'like is cured by like': the substance that can cause the symptoms in a healthy person can cure the same symptoms in a sick person (Trevelyan and Booth 1994). Homoeopathic medicines are prescribed on the basis of a holistic review of the patient's condition (Wilkinson 2002).

Research

Contrary to popular belief there is a wealth of research covering a wide range of therapies. The body of knowledge, according to CAM, is one that is forever expanding (Mantle 1999). There remains, however, a lack of scientific evidence to prove the efficacy and safety of complementary medicine. This was highlighted in the discussion document *Integrated Healthcare: A way forward for the next five years?* (Foundation for Integrated Medicine 1998), which noted that there was little high-quality and appropriate research (and capacity) into the safety, efficacy and effectiveness of CAM. Concerns were also expressed about the dilemma that the general public faced when seeking an appropriate treatment that could be helpful, appropriate and safe for their particular condition. The Royal London Homoeopathic Hospital (1999) highlights reasons for the limited research into complementary therapies, such as lack of financial resources, inadequate research skills and academic infrastructure, and finally, lack of patients to substantiate research. Penson (1998), conversely, argues that part of the difficulty in researching this topic is the result of the complexity of adopting a holistic approach.

In 2002, initiated by the Prince of Wales Foundation for Integrated Health as part of its research strategy for CAM, the Alternative and Complementary Collaborative for Research and Development (ACCoRD) was established. Representatives on the group are professionals from acupuncture, chiropractic, herbal medicine, homoeopathy, nutritional therapy, naturopathy, osteopathy and reflexology, in addition to representation from professional bodies – the Royal College of Nursing and the Complementary Therapies in Nursing Forum. The aim of the foundation is the development of high-quality, relevant research into the safety, effectiveness, patient satisfaction and efficacy of all forms of health care, especially those therapies regarded as complementary. Information dissemination is proposed through a programme of conferences and seminars (Anon 2002).

Tavares (2003) notes that a lack of evidence in some therapies does not necessarily mean a lack of effectiveness. It is apparent from information acquired from the numerous studies undertaken that patients clearly value complementary therapies.

Conclusion

Since the 1980s there has been an increasing integration of complementary therapies within mainstream health services (Mantle 1997). A holistic approach to treatment, which considers their physical, mental and spiritual well-being, is patient driven and continues to increase. This is further acknowledged in the foreword written by HRH the Prince of Wales in the *National Guidelines for the Use of Complementary Therapies in Supportive and Palliative Care* (Tavares 2003).

These guidelines have been written for managers and those responsible for the development of complementary services and aim to 'provide information and recommend activities which can contribute to quality improvement, patient safety and improved outcomes' (Tavares 2003, p. 11).

They also seek to address issues directly related to patient safety and the provision of complementary services, such as clinical governance, regulation, training of therapists, audit and evaluation (Tavares 2003, p. 6). Palliative and cancer care are paramount in the production of this document and a resource for those involved with service development.

Health professionals are in a key position to integrate complementary therapies within clinical practice; the competence and knowledge to assess the appropriateness of each therapy are essential. Heightened awareness

of the benefits, risks and patient safety is the responsibility of professionals as accountable practitioners (UKCC 1992a, 1992b, section 6.1).

Summary of key points

- Cancer patients are turning more and more towards complementary
  therapies.
- Within the NHS in the UK, almost all cancer centres, hospice and palliative
  care units offer some form of complementary therapy.
- Nurses are in a key position to incorporate complementary therapies into
  practice. As accountable practitioners, they must be aware of their
  responsibility to patients.
- In 2003 The Prince of Wales Foundation of Integrated Medicine published
  guidelines for the use of complementary therapies in supportive and
  palliative care.
- The Prince of Wales Foundation reviewed nine therapies widely used in palliative and supportive care for their perceived beneficial effects; these
  include: massage, aromatherapy, reflexology, reiki, spiritual healing,
  therapeutic touch, hypnosis, hypnotherapy, acupuncture and homoeopathy.
- Further research is needed into the risks and benefits of complementary
  therapies.

References

Anon (2002) News update. Foundation for Integrated Medicine in Complementary Therapies
in Nursing and Midwifery 6: 56-8.
Arcier M (1990) Aromatherapy. London: Hamlyn.
Beech N (2001) Complementary therapies. In: Corner J, Bailey B (eds), Cancer Nursing Care
in Context. London: Blackwell Science.
Brewer J (1989) Alternative approach-profile. Nursing Standard 3(50): 46.
British Medical Acupuncture Society (2003) www.medical-acupuncture.co.uk/code.pdf.
Byers D (1983). Better Health with Foot Reflexology. USA: Ingram Publishing, Inc.
Calvert R (2003) A new image for the old adage. In: Tavares M (ed.), National Guidelines for
the Use of Complementary Therapies in Supportive and Palliative Care. London: The
Prince of Wales Foundation for Integrated Health.
Cawthorn A, Carter A (2000) Aromatherapy and its application in cancer and palliative care.
Complementary Therapies in Nursing and Midwifery 6: 83-6.
Corner J, Bailey B (eds) (2001) Cancer Nursing Care in Context. London: Blackwell Science.
De Valois B (2003) Aromatherapy for people with cancer. In Essence 2(1): 22-6.
Douglas D (2003) Explaining hypnotherapy. Avon Hypnotherapy:
www.avonhyponotherapy.co.uk.
Egan EC (1992) Therapeutic touch. In: Snyder I (ed.), Independent Nursing Interventions. New
York: Delmar Publishers, Inc.
Ernst E (1999) House of Lords' Select Committee on Science and Technology - Sixth Report:
www.parliament.the-stationery-office.co.uk.

Expert Advisory Group on Cancer (1995) The Calman–Hine Report: A policy framework for commissioning cancer services. London: The Stationery Office.

Feigel RW, Victors I, Zollman A et al. (2000) Cited in Tavares (2003).

Foundation for Integrated Medicine (1998) Integrated Healthcare: A way forward for the next five years? A discussion document. London: Foundation for Integrated Medicine.

Fulder SJ (1988) Complementary therapies. In: Corner J, Bailey B (eds), Cancer Nursing Care in Context. London: Blackwell Science.

Furnham A (1996) Why do people use complementary therapies? In: Ernst E (ed.), Complementary Therapies: An objective appraisal. London: Butterworth-Heineman.

Gray RA (2000) The use of massage therapy in palliative care. Complementary Therapies in Nursing and Midwifery 6: 77-82.

Jackson AJ (2003) Massage therapy. In: Tavares M (ed.), National Guidelines for the Use of Complementary Therapies in Supportive and Palliative Care. London: Prince of Wales Foundation for Integrated Medicine.

Kassab S, Stevenson C (1996) Common misunderstandings about complementary therapies for patients with cancer. Complementary Therapies in Nursing and Midwifery 2: 62-5.

Krieger D (1975) The theory and practice of therapeutic touch. In: Sayre-Adams J, Wright S (eds), Therapeutic Touch. Edinburgh: Churchill Livingstone.

Lewith M (2002) Cited in Tavares (2003).

Lidell L, Thomas S, Cooke CB (eds) (1990) The Book of Massage: The complete step-by-step guide to eastern and western techniques. Edinburgh: Ebury Press.

Lynn J (1996) National occupational standards for reflexology. Moving experiences. Nursing Times 92(14): 46-8.

Macmillan Cancer Relief (2002) The Directory of Complementary Therapy Services in UK Cancer Care. London: Macmillan Cancer Relief.

McNamara P (1997) Massage for people with cancer. The use of massage therapy in palliative care. Complementary Therapies in Nursing and Midwifery 6: 77-82.

McVey MLV-T (2000) Policy development. Complementary Therapies in Nursing and Midwifery 6: 50-5.

Mantle F (1997) Implementing evidence in practice. British Journal of Community Health Nursing 2(1): 36-9.

Mantle F (1999) Complementary Therapies: Is there an evidence base? London: Emap Healthcare Ltd.

Maxwell-Hudson C (1990) Introduction. In: Lidell L, Thomas S, Cooke CB (eds), The Book of Massage: The complete step-by-step guide to eastern and western techniques. Edinburgh: Ebury Press.

Montague A (1986) Cited in Price and Price (1995).

National Federation of Spiritual Healers (1998) www.nfsh.org.uk

National Federation of Spiritual Healers (2003) www.nfsh.org.uk

Norman L, Cowan T (1988) The Reflexology Handbook: A complete guide. Avon: The Bath Press.

Penson J (1998) Complementary therapies: making a difference in palliative care. Complementary Therapies in Nursing and Midwifery 4: 77-81.

Price S (1985) Aromatherapy Training Notes. Hinkley, Leics: International College of Aromatherapy.

Price S, Price L (1995) Aromatherapy for Health Professionals. Edinburgh: Churchill Livingstone.

Prince of Wales Foundation for Integrated Health (2003) A Guide to Our Work. London: POWFIH.

Rankin-Box D (1996) Focus on complementary therapies. British Journal of Community Health Nursing 2(1): 25-9.

Royal London Homoeopathic Hospital (1999) The Evidence Base of Complementary Medicine. 2nd edn. London: Causeway Communications.

Stevenson C (1997) Complementary therapies: education for community practice. British Journal of Community Health Nursing 2(1): 30-4.

Stone J (1999) Using complementary therapies within nursing: some ethical and legal considerations. Complementary Therapies in Nursing and Midwifery 5: 46-50.

Tavares M (ed.) (2003) National Guidelines for the Use of Complementary Therapies in Supportive and Palliative Care. London: Prince of Wales Foundation for Integrated Health.

Tissarand R, Balacs T (1995) Essential Oil Safety. A guide for health care professionals. London: Churchill Livingstone.

Trevelyan J, Booth B (1994) Complementary Medicine for Nurses, Midwives and Health Visitors. London: Macmillan Press.

Tue A (1999) Acupuncture. In: Gao D (ed.), The Encyclopaedia of Chinese Medicine. Surrey: Carlton Books Ltd.

United Kingdom Central Council (1992a) Scope of Professional Practice. London: UKCC.

United Kingdom Central Council (1992b) Standards for the Administration of Medicines, Section 39. London: UKCC.

Weil A, Rees L (2001) Integrated medicine. Complementary medicine. British Medical Journal 322: 119-20.

West R (1994) Alternative medicine: prospects and speculations. In: Trevelyan J, Booth B (eds), Complementary Medicine for Nurses, Midwives and Health Visitors. London: Macmillan Press.

Wilkinson S (2002) Complementary therapies patient demand. International Journal of Palliative Nursing 8: 468.

Wright S (2004) Hard to measure. Nursing Standard 18(23): 24.

World Health Organization (1986) Health for All by the Year 2000: Charter for action. Geneva: WHO.

Chapter 14

Help and support for cancer patients and their families

Rose Amey

Support from a professional social worker for patients and their families can be very beneficial. This chapter explores the type of social work assistance available for patients with colorectal cancer and their carers.

Framework

Social work is associated with the provision of services; in practice, services are offered only to select groups, who are frequently referred to as vulnerable adults. People usually considered within this category are those who experience disability, long-term illness or frailty, resulting in an inability to care for themselves, or those who have insufficient understanding of their own needs to enable them to live safely, possibly in immediate danger of exploitation, and in some cases those who pose a risk to other people (Johns 2003).

Referral by the health-care professional for social work support can be helpful to the colorectal cancer patient. Social workers are trained to deal with human interaction whether that interaction is between a person and her or his self-image, the person and other people, the person and her or his environment, or a combination of these factors. Using social work skills, guided discussion with individuals and families enables some service users to resolve their own problems, overcome fears and anxieties, and re-affirm their normal coping capacity (Coulshed 1988). Others may need support to access appropriate services and sources of advice or provision (Hadley et al. 1987).

The social worker is the creation of statute (Brayne and Martin 2001). The Local Authority Social Services Act 1970 requires local authorities to establish a Social Services Committee to administer Social Service functions, which are exercised under the general supervision of the Secretary of State. Working within a very strict legal framework (Table 14.1) and carrying a caseload of service users to whom they have a statutory duty, relationships are established with each individual service user. This enables the social worker to act as an advocate if necessary, permitting service users' wishes to prevail.

Table 14.1 Legislation

Primary legislation

Carers (Recognition and Services) Act 1995
Carers and Disabled Children Act 2000
Chronically Sick and Disabled Persons Act 1970
Community Care (Direct Payments) Act 1996
Community Care (Residential Accommodation) Act 1998
Data Protection Act 1998
Disability Discrimination Act 1995
Disability Rights Commission Act 1999
Disabled Persons (Services, Consultation and Representation) Act 1986
Enduring Power of Attorney Act 1985
Mental Health Act 1983
National Health Service and Community Care Act 1990
Protection of Children Act 1999
Race Relations Act 1976
Race Relations Amendment Act 2000

Secondary Legislation

Data Protection (Subject Access Modification) (Social Work) Order 2000

Additional information about the legislative framework informing social work practice can be obtained from Brayne and Marsh (2001).

There is no specific law that promotes empowerment; however, there is legislation promoting rights. The Race Relations Act 1976 and the Race Relations Amendment Act 2000 are anti-discriminatory legislation that need the endorsement of good race relations. The social worker shows an understanding of oppressive processes such as institutional discrimination, demonstrates awareness and understanding of oppression and the challenges of working proactively with diversity. In addition, recognition of cultural issues, gender and colour-blind perspectives (Dominelli 1988), and respect for the emotional and spiritual needs, are an integral part of any assessment.

An understanding of the Mental Health Act 1983 informs practice for service users who in addition to colorectal cancer have a mental health problem. The Disabled Persons (Services, Consultation and Representation) Act 1986, the Disability Discrimination Act 1995 and the Disability Rights Commission Act 1999 include anti-discriminatory law and the right to advocacy for disabled people, another group who could be disadvantaged by an additional problem such as a diagnosis of colorectal cancer.

The Chronically Sick and Disabled Persons Act 1970 and the National Health Service (NHS) and Community Care Act 1990 impose on local authorities, normally the employers of social workers, a duty to provide information about services. These services vary from area to area; equally the individual cost levied by the local authority differs. In addition to knowledge of locally provided statutory services, the social worker has knowledge about voluntary and charitable agency networks within the locality that can offer support. Access to other information includes national charities, and sources of support and advice. Social Services departments frequently employ a welfare rights worker, who can assist users to negotiate the welfare benefits system, a very complex area, which may offer financial support for service users and their families who have a loss of income, or a change in role status caused by the diagnosis of cancer. Frequently used helpline numbers are listed in Resources at the end of the chapter.

The NHS and Community Care Act 1990 offers users the right to assessment of needs; however, local authorities cannot impose these services. There is no obligation to act in the best interests of an adult, unlike the responsibility to a child (Protection of Children Act 1999). Any assessment has to centre on need; currently there are plans for a single assessment tool enabling a multiprofessional contribution, the aim being to provide a seamless service. Assessment has to be conducted before a decision is made about what services, if any, are to be offered, not determined by availability. The social worker has ongoing responsibility for monitoring the relevance and effectiveness of any services implemented. The Community Care (Direct Payments) Act 1996 gives every user the right to choose and recompense their service provider.

The Carers and Disabled Children Act 2000 and/or Carers (Recognition and Services) Act 1995 offers every carer the right to an independent assessment of his or her current and prospective ability to care for someone, giving consideration to ways in which they can be supported in this role.

Mindful consideration of the Data Protection Act 1998 underlines the legal requirement to share information with the service user; social workers have a general duty, in common law, to safeguard the confidentiality of personal information. There are clear limitations on the extent of confidentiality; in principle information can be shared only by agreement; however, in circumstances where there is a risk of harm to others, disclosure is the social worker's responsibility.

Intervention

Social workers have a long history of multidisciplinary team working for the benefit of patients in a wide variety of settings, collaborating with other professional groups as part of the social work process (Thompson 2000). Effective functioning, which is most beneficial to both patient and her or his family, occurs in an atmosphere where there is trust and respect within the multidisciplinary team (Badawi and Biamonti 1990). *The NHS Cancer Plan* indicates a requirement for effective multidisciplinary team-working to advantage patients (Department of Health 2000).

It is not everyone who needs referral to a social worker during his or her journey through ill-health and the medical system, but there are a number of occasions when this should be given consideration. The following situations are broadly suggested: at the time of diagnosis; when a choice is necessary about a programme of treatment; the planning phase of hospital discharge; and disease recurrence, when a decision has been made to offer palliative care.

Diagnosis

At diagnosis an assessment of the concerned social factors can offer an essential contribution at an emotionally charged time. For many the diagnosis of colorectal cancer will come as a shock; for others it confirms their suspicions; some may have been unwell and unable to work for some time, others may have endured a period of 'tests'. For many the news will come at a time that is potentially difficult for a wide variety of social reasons. Assistance and advice enabling the patient and her or his family to maximize their own resources, together with consideration of other areas of support that may be available to them, can enable embarkation upon a treatment plan with a greater sense of security. Social workers can facilitate patients to develop strategies for both obtaining information and retaining information in a medical setting, which can otherwise seem daunting (Buckman 1995).

Issues affecting the social welfare of patients and families can include employment, child care, care of elderly dependants, finances, especially existing debts, welfare benefits already in payment or which may now be applicable, insurance, mortgages, housing, travel costs for treatment or the family to visit, and a patient's own personal or domestic care needs. Other concerns where the social worker is trained to offer support may include maintenance of family role, body image and issues around sexuality.

Treatment

Decisions on the best method of treatment for colorectal cancer where alternative options are available can depend equally on social and medical considerations. Medical services may be ineffective, or less beneficial if they are delivered without consideration for the patient's way of life and potential social adaptation. A social worker can act as a patient advocate to enable treatment to be offered in a way that is the least demanding socially or financially. This is of immense importance when therapy is offered over a protracted period, or at some distance from a patient's home. Those patients on low income, or who have active caring responsibilities or pre-existing medical problem(s), can experience considerable difficulty during prolonged periods of therapy. Many lack the necessary self-confidence or articulacy to negotiate treatment attendance times, and may feel that they should be grateful for any treatment offered.

Discharge preparation and ongoing support

Discharge from hospital can also be a very stressful time for some cancer patients (see also Chapters 9 and 10). At this stage they may feel weak, lacking in confidence following surgical procedures, or are adjusting to a temporary or permanent colostomy and feel immobilized by body image changes. Diagnosis and intervention may have followed in rapid succession, leaving feelings of shock and disorientation. Timely discussion with a social worker, ideally not at the point of discharge from hospital, about plans for coping at home can enable the patient and family to consider their own resources. If necessary social workers can assist with provision of statutory or voluntary support, for a period of rehabilitation, or longer if appropriate. Liaison with other disciplines such as an occupational therapist is frequently enlisted, within either a social services department or a medical setting, to facilitate assessment for, and provision of, aids for daily living, including small items such as helping hands and perching stools, to larger items including wheelchairs and stair lifts. Occupational therapists employed by social service departments also assist with grant applications for major adaptations to service users' homes in situations where deemed necessary.

Disease recurrence

Recurrence of colorectal cancer is an extremely emotionally charged time and some patients often feel the need to pause and consider their options; it is a time when personal resources need to be re-charged to address the future. Many patients require a social worker to listen while considering issues around failure, and whose failure it is. Others may have exhausted their physical, emotional and financial assets while encountering cancer for the first time, and want assistance to revisit local and national support provision.

If ongoing care is considered palliative, social workers are equipped to offer assistance, with the amelioration of emotional and practical difficulties previously addressed during the disease process (Oliviere et al. 1987), thus enabling a patient to gain quality and control through the remaining period of life. It may be necessary during this final stage of life to help patients plan their dependants' ongoing care by facilitating the introduction of a legal adviser to assist with a will or other legal documents, such as power of attorney (Enduring Power of Attorney Act 1985). There are times when guidance is required with funeral arrangements or assistance with referral to a spiritual adviser, particularly in those patients whose belief is considered unconventional.

Social work training includes the development of listening skills, enabling them to be supportive emotionally and practically at the end-stage of the disease process. Sensitivity at this time can mean that death is remembered by the bereaved in a more positive way. Provision of appropriate non-intrusive services, which offer practical relief to patients, families and significant others at this very private time, can be indispensable. This kind of support may also be appreciated by other professionals who offer care, including general practitioners and community and specialist nurses.

Patients diagnosed with colorectal cancer who have an existing medical problem and who are established service users, may find that they are entitled to additional assistance to meet their current need. Similarly welfare benefits, whether they are already being received, or because of the cancer diagnosis, will need assessment. Those patients who have a sensory loss or a learning disability may also benefit from a social worker referral for similar reasons. This also applies to patients who live in residential/nursing care homes, who, irrespective of their financial status, could be entitled to additional health authority contributions towards the cost of care.

Recent legislation, the Community Care (Delayed Discharges etc.) Act 2003, which relates to patients being discharged from hospital who need care, will also have implications for those with colorectal cancer. This legislation removes the local authority's power to charge for certain community care services, and imposes a specified number of days to put together a discharge plan for service users leaving an acute hospital. Under this new legislation the local authority is required to make a payment to the relevant NHS organization when it has not been possible to arrange services for those patients whose assessment fulfilled the recognized criteria for support.

Conclusion

To summarize, the input of a professional social worker to enable patients, their carers and significant others can ameliorate many of the problems experienced throughout the cancer journey to ongoing and terminal care. Their competencies include listening skills, an understanding of human growth and development, individual and group behaviour, family dynamics and issues arising from role change. Other responsibilities include consideration of diversity, and updated knowledge of local/national resources, both voluntary and statutory. The inclusion of a social worker to support patients with colorectal cancer can also add a positive and interesting aspect to the multidisciplinary team.

Summary of key points

Social workers have a multifaceted role which includes:

- Multidisciplinary team work.
- Support and at times acting as patient advocate.
- Training and the development of interpersonal skills.
- Access to a range of community-based services to assist patient/carers practically and emotionally.
- Assisting patients to plan their care and the ongoing care of any dependants.

References

Badawi M, Biamonti B (1990) Social Work Practice in Health Care. Cambridge: Woodhead Faulkner.

Brayne M, Marsh G (2001) Law for Social Workers. Basingstoke: Macmillan.

Buckman R (1995) What You Really Need To Know About Cancer. London: Key Porter Books, in collaboration with Macmillan Cancer Relief.

Coulshed V (1988) Social Work Practice: An introduction. Basingstoke: Macmillan.

Department of Health (2000) The NHS Cancer Plan: A plan for investment, a plan for reform. London: HMSO.

Dominelli L (1988) Anti-Racist Social Work. Basingstoke: Macmillan.

Hadley R, Cooper M, Dale P et al. (1987) A Community Social Workers' Handbook. London: Tavistock Publications.

Harland S, Griffiths D (2001) A Guide to Grants for Individuals in Need. London: Directory of Social Change.

Johns R (2003) Using The Law in Social Work. Exeter: Learning Matters.

Oliviere D, Hargeaves R, Monroe B (1987) Good Practices in Palliative Care. London: Ashgate Arena.

Thompson N (2000) Understanding Social Work: Preparing for practice. Basingstoke: Macmillan.

Useful reading

Department of Health (2003) A Practical Guide for Disabled People or Carers. London: Department of Health.

Donaghey V, Bernal J, Tuffrey-Wijne I et al. (2002) Getting on with Cancer: Books beyond words series. London: Gaskell/St George's Medical School.

Greaves I (2003–2004) Disability Rights Handbook. London: Disability Alliance.

Rios C (ed.) (2002) Charities Digest. London: Waterlow Professional Publishing.

Thompson N (2000) Understanding Social Work Preparing for Practice. Basingstoke: Macmillan.

Resources

Sources of help and support

Action Cancer: 028 9080 3344
Beating Bowel Cancer: 020 8892 5256
Bristol Cancer Help Centre: 0117 980 9505
British Colostomy Association: 0800 328 4257
CancerBACUP: 0808 800 1234
Cancer Black Care: 020 7249 1097
Carers UK: 020 7566 7602
Crocus Trust: 0870 242 4870 (disseminates information about the symptoms
   of bowel cancer)
Cruse – Bereavement Care: 020 8940 4818
GaysCan helpline: 020 8368 9027
Ileostomy and Internal Pouch Association: 01724 720150
Macmillan Cancer Relief: 0808 808 2020
Marie Curie Cancer Care: 0800 716146
National Cancer Alliance: 01865 793566
Tenovus Cancer Information Centre: 0808 808 1010; www.ican4u.com

Additional

Age Concern, Astral house, 1268 London Road, London SW16 4ER.
   Tel: 020 8679 8000
British Association of Sexual and Marital Therapy, PO Box 62,
   Sheffield S10 3TS
Impotence Information Centre, PO Box 1130, London W3 9BB
The Patient Association, PO Box 935, Harrow, Middlesex HA1 3YJ.
   Tel: 020 8423 8999
Relate, Herbert Gray College, Little Church Street, Rugby CV21 3AP.
   Tel: 01788 573241
Samaritans, 10 The Grove, Slough SL1 1QP. Tel: 0345 909090

Index

Page numbers in **bold type** refer to figure; those in *italics* to tables